The
Reverse
Diet

The Reverse Diet

Lose 20, 50, 100 Pounds
or More by Eating
Dinner for Breakfast
and Breakfast for Dinner

TRICIA CUNNINGHAM
AND
HEIDI SKOLNIK, MS, CDN

BICENTENNIAL
1807
WILEY
2007
BICENTENNIAL

John Wiley & Sons, Inc.

Published by John Wiley & Sons, Inc., Hoboken, New Jersey
Published simultaneously in Canada

Design and composition by Navta Associates, Inc.

The information contained in this book is not intended to serve as a replacement for professional medical advice. Any use of the information in this book is at the reader's discretion. The author and the publisher specifically disclaim any and all liability arising directly or indirectly from the use or application of any information contained in this book. A health care professional should be consulted regarding your specific situation.

For general information about our other products and services, please contact our Customer Care Department within the United States at (800) 762-2974, outside the United States at (317) 572-3993 or fax (317) 572-4002.

Wiley also publishes its books in a variety of electronic formats. Some content that appears in print may not be available in electronic books. For more information about Wiley products, visit our web site at www.wiley.com.

Library of Congress Cataloging-in-Publication Data:

Cunningham, Tricia, date.
    The reverse diet : lose 20, 50, 100 pounds or more by eating dinner for breakfast and breakfast for dinner / Tricia Cunningham and Heidi Skolnik.
        p. cm.
    Includes index.
    ISBN-13 978-0-470-05229-7 (cloth)
    ISBN-10 0-470-05229-5 (cloth)
    1. Reducing diets. 2. Food portions. 3. Food habits. I. Skolnik, Heidi, 1961- II. Title.
    RM222.2.C86 2006
    613.2'5—dc22
                                                                    2006025135

Printed in the United States of America

10 9 8 7 6 5 4 3 2 1

This book is dedicated to all Reverse Dieters who have committed themselves to becoming happier and healthier individuals. To my daughters, Brittni and Noelle, for all you have endured and for bringing the greatest joy to my life. And to Sean, my best friend, partner, husband, and one true love.

—Tricia

To Jinny Skolnik and Arthur Skolnik (in loving memory), who fed me three square meals a day plus snacks along with healthy doses of support, delight, encouragement, an emphasis on education, and an appreciation of hard work.

—Heidi

CONTENTS

Acknowledgments   ix

Tricia's Story   1

Heidi's Story   6

Introduction   9

PART ONE
The Reverse Diet Weight-Loss Phase

1 What Is the Reverse Diet?   17

2 The Reverse Diet Food List and Reverse Diet Basics   30

3 Reverse Diet Meal Plans and Meal Planning   49

4 Reverse Diet Portions—and Plateaus   78

5 Reverse Diet Motivation: Dealing with High-Risk
       Moments   88

PART TWO
The Reverse Diet Bridge Phase

6 The Reverse Diet Bridge Food List and Meal Plans   123

7 The Reverse Diet Accelerated: Building Lean Muscle
       and More   150

PART THREE
The Reverse Diet Maintenance Phase

8 The Reverse Diet for Life   171

9 Reverse Diet Recipes   185

Appendix A Food Reality Check   239

Appendix B Calcium Sources   244

Appendix C The Six Food Groups and Servings   246

Index   249

ACKNOWLEDGMENTS

When I began my Reverse Diet journey, it never dawned on me that it would lead me to where we are today—holding this book. There have been many hills and valleys over these past seven years, and bringing this book to life has been like climbing Mount Everest. With that said, I would like to thank those who have guided me, walked with me, and climbed with me, and who sometimes had to pull me up that ferocious mountain: My husband, Sean, who knows me better than anyone and has my heart and soul. If there was ever a marriage whose vows for better or for worse, for richer or for poorer, in sickness and in health were tested to the max, it was ours. Thank you for hanging in there every time I said, "Just two more weeks." My girls, Brittni and Noelle, the most beautiful, loving and gifted creatures on Earth. To Chad, the son I always prayed for. I admire you all beyond words, and I love you. To my late grandparents, Pat and Bob, for your wisdom, love, security, and all those years you allowed me to entertain you in your living room holding a brush for a microphone. Thanks to my mum, and to my two dads, who watched me melt before their eyes, and for their love, support, and always being there and showing me that dreams really can come true. And my brother, Chris, who I know will never be anywhere in this world without *The Reverse Diet* in his hand.

Thank you, *Good Morning America*, especially Diane Sawyer, the producers, and Lemita Fields, for truly hearing what I had to say and introducing Heidi and me. I feel truly blessed to have Heidi as a huge part of this book—thank you. Hayden Meyer of UTA, who saw something special in me and signed me on to my new life. Wendy Bell, of WTAE in Pittsburgh, for bringing my story to life and to the public for the first time. *First for Women* magazine for introducing the face of the Reverse Dieter. *Woman's World*, who made me feel like a glamour girl for a day. Anna Lang for believing in the Reverse Diet and more important herself. To all of the members of the Reverse Diet Support Group, the Sunshine Club, for your commitment, motivation, sharing your struggles and successes, and your true passion of helping others. Kudos to all who ever have been a part of my life, for you have helped shape me into the person I am today.

—Tricia

To Bradley, who fuels me with his very being. A huge thank you coupled with appreciation for all the help and opportunities along the way to: Michelle Cole, David Weiss, Jane Purcell, Allen Lans, George Bardis, Ronnie Barnes and the Giants Organization, Pete Libman and SAB, Lisa Callahan, Jo Hannafin, Terry Karl and the Women's Sports Medicine Center at Hospital for Special Surgery, Mike Motta, Lewis Maharam, Lou Schuller, Karen Mazzota and *Men's Health* magazine, Bonnie Block, Jim Motzer, Lucy Danziger, Mike O'Shea, and Abbey Corsum Sims. To Lewis (and family) who has moved from mentor to friend.

To Judith Belasco for helping with research; Lisa Adler, MS, RD, for patience and tenacity in analyzing menus and recipes; and Andrea Chernus, MS, RD. To Fran Einhorn for her input into the cover and organization and Julie for always showing up when I needed extra help.

And finally to my circle of friends and family without whom I would be unable to destress (and then be left to overeat): Tata and the rest of the Weitzmans; the Goldberg, Zweibach, Hubbel, Goetz, Sable, and Scherr families; and Neil (still). To Dan, Renee, Wendy,

Michele, Julie, Stacey, Charlee, Eve, Stacey, Mark and Max, Doug, Peter, Maryanne, Robin, Jamie and Shelly, Lori Lynn, Tom, Daron, Dianne and Ron, Jeff, Melorra, Robyn, Larry, Mary Kay, Ken, Marcy, and last, but not at all least, Fred.

—Heidi

Tom Miller, Juliet Grames, Lisa Burstiner, and Kerry Weinstein at Wiley for your belief in this book. To Joe Regal, Lauren, and Peter for your faith, insight, and devotion to this project. A special thank you from our hearts goes to Michael Psaltis and Bess Reed for being not only two terrific agents but great friends. Michael, we would choose you to be our advocate anytime!

The granddaddy thank you goes to the hardest-working, devoted, and artistic writer, editor, and friend we know: Amy Hughes, you have a wonderful passion for what you do, and you do it well.

—Heidi and Tricia

Tricia's Story

One day six years ago, I woke up and decided to do exactly the opposite of what I had been doing my whole life. Up until that point, I had spent most of my life struggling with a weight problem. I yo-yoed between bingeing and fasting and eventually tipped the scale at 280 pounds on a 5'8" frame.

Until that time, even throughout my childhood, I thought nothing of being 150 to 160 pounds. I wasn't one of the thin girls. My weight became a way for me to protect myself from the abuse I suffered at home. If I made myself ugly, I figured that I was less of a target for my first stepfather's unwelcome attention. Even though I eventually moved to live with my grandmother, this habit stuck with me. Fear of being attractive created a lifelong struggle with my weight.

My weight fluctuated for many years. I tried everything, including starvation and just about every fad diet, all of which failed miserably. Ultimately I gained more weight than I lost. Nothing seemed to work. My family tried to convince me that I was "big-boned" and that there was nothing I could do about it. But when I married my first husband, Ron, at age nineteen, he didn't accept that logic. He wanted me to be super-thin, and he wasn't patient. I was back to starving myself and binge eating. By Christmas 1991 I managed to get down to a size 9 and felt great. Valentine's Day 1992 came with a special surprise: I was pregnant with my first child, Brittni. Of course I welcomed this blessing, but it presented a whole new challenge.

Having struggled with weight all my life and then being told that I had to gain weight, I was in an emotional whirlwind. I thought I had a free pass to eat whatever I wanted. Ron worked as a supervisor for a local snack food company, and just about every night he brought home as many snacks as he could carry. Three-pound bags of potato chips, Slim Jims, cookies—you name it. I was in heaven. At the end of the pregnancy in October 1992, I weighed 220 pounds, having gained 70 pounds. After I had Brittni, my eating habits didn't go back to the way they had been before the pregnancy and therefore neither did my weight. In March 1993, I learned I was pregnant with my second child. I was delighted, and once again I had a free pass to eat whatever I wanted.

Not long after Noelle was born, Ron was back on the subject of my weight. He hounded me about not losing weight after having Brittni. He was constantly comparing me to a woman in his office and complaining that I wasn't nearly as skinny as she was. It didn't take long before I realized they were having an affair, and soon after that my marriage with Ron dissolved. Over the next few years, I had a few short romantic relationships, and my weight would fluctuate accordingly. Bingeing and starving were my two best friends. I ate a lot during stressful times and nothing after I had done something wrong—that is, anything less than perfect. I was a perfectionist and an overachiever in all aspects of life except where my weight was concerned. That was the one thing I felt I couldn't control.

I was the heaviest I had ever been, maxing out at 292 pounds. I kept starving myself and losing as much as 40 pounds, but it always came back. I just couldn't keep the weight off.

Then on August 28, 1999, everything changed. I woke up exhausted from a party the night before. We had been celebrating the life of a friend we'd lost, and I was still dealing with my emotions as I slowly made my way downstairs. I moved slowly because I was wearing a cast on my right leg, which I had broken a few weeks earlier during a tumble down the steps. I couldn't see my feet over my belly, tripped, and went flying. It was nine-thirty in the morning and the house was crowded with people over to watch a sporting event. We ordered a pizza, and I had my usual drink, Caffeine-Free Diet Pepsi, along with my morning cigarette—I was smoking two and a half packs a day. Everything seemed normal. After four puffs of my cigarette, three bites of pizza, and a half a glass of my drink, my heart felt like it was getting ready to burst. Everything was spinning out of control; it felt like there was a swarm of bees in my head, and I dropped everything and ran into the bathroom.

I was suffering from the worst panic attack I had ever experienced. As a trained nurse, I knew what to do; I started running my wrists under cold water, but that didn't work. My daughters were trying to talk me down. Even so, my heart was racing. The girls ran a cold bath for me, and I soaked in it for two hours. I still didn't feel right. I was afraid to go to a doctor; I feared that something awful was happening. The attack went on for the next five hours before finally subsiding. I went back into the bathroom and looked in the mirror. I hated what I saw; I hated myself. There I was with two beautiful daughters, years of education, and the world in front of me, and I was killing myself, destroying my body, and ruining my future.

After the panic attack, I tried to figure out what had brought it on. I thought it must have been something I ate, drank, or smoked, so I refused to eat or drink for the rest of the day (and I have never had another cigarette). I did not eat or drink anything for the next three days. On the fourth morning, I woke up and knew that I couldn't keep starving myself. I looked into the mirror and didn't hate what I saw, because I began to realize that I could change it. I knew that everything I had done up to that point with my weight and health had been wrong. I knew that I couldn't keep living the way I was living. I had to reverse course—to flip-flop everything—to change my life. That was the beginning of the Reverse Diet.

I went into the kitchen that fourth morning extremely hungry, but still frightened from the panic attack and worried that food would cause another attack. I stuck to basic ingredients, nothing exotic. The first breakfast included a plain chicken breast, a baked potato, and some broccoli. No butter, spices, or salt. I took my time, checking my pulse every few minutes. Everything seemed fine, and I felt good. Within a couple of hours, I was hungry again, so for lunch I had more chicken and veggies. My belly always growled by dinner-time, as it was the only big meal I typically had, but this day there was no growling. I wasn't hungry and ate very little: just a small serving of plain, dry, shredded wheat. The next morning I was very hungry, so I ate the same things because I knew they were safe. For the next week, I continued the same routine: my dinner in the morning, a smaller meal for lunch, and a small breakfast for dinner. I saw that my clothes were getting loose and I was shedding a few pounds, but I didn't know that I had lost 12 pounds in a week! By the time I got my cast off in September, just a month later, I had lost 40 pounds.

I started to think that something was wrong with me—there was no way I could eat that much food every day and lose weight without something being wrong. While I definitely watched the foods I ate, my meals weren't tiny and unsatisfying as they had been on every diet I had ever been on. Instead, I ate until I was full. How do you lose weight by eating more? This didn't make sense to me. I made an appointment with my doctor, who did a complete physical and told me that I was entirely healthy—in fact, healthier than I had ever been. I couldn't believe my ears. Not only was I not dying, I was actually going to live longer. I became obsessed with the concept of *eat more food, lose more weight*. I bought diet book after diet book, searching for the answers to my questions, but I was on my own. I'd have to figure this out by myself.

Some of the changes to my lifestyle I just fell into. It started with me trying to have the fewest ingredients for a light dinner. I chose cereal (shredded wheat), but I didn't want the milk. I used to drink orange juice every morning, so one day I just decided to mix it in. I know shredded wheat with orange juice sounds weird, but I really liked it, plus it satisfied my sweet craving. Other aspects of the plan took research and experimentation.

That New Year's Eve, I went to a party wearing a size 9 dress. I had gone from 250 pounds in August down to just 150 pounds. I had set a goal weight of 130 pounds and knew that I could reach it. By March 2000, I was at 130. I even got as low as 112, but that was too thin for my build. I went back to 130 and have stayed that weight ever since. Now I work as a motivational coach for fellow Reverse Dieters and have dedicated my life to helping others reverse their lives the same way I did. All that I have learned is in the pages that follow. I have teamed up with Heidi Skolnik, a knowledgeable nutritionist, and together we've made this diet something that can work for everyone.

Heidi's Story

I love food and enjoy eating. As a nutritionist, I work with people every day to help them understand how good nutrition can help them feel better, think better, perform better, and live better and perhaps longer. I believe that daily activity coupled with healthful eating goes a long way in improving the quality of our lives. I can't help my clients with their finances, child care, elder care, or communication skills, but I can lessen the physiological stress of poor eating and poor physical fitness that ultimately plays a role in life's challenges.

I am fond of chocolate and ice cream, especially vanilla ice cream with chocolate chips. Many people don't think that a nutritionist would ever eat such things, but that's a big misconception. When I meet people, they often say things like, "Oh, you probably never eat anything bad for you because you're a nutritionist." But I do! Along with eating foods that are less than nutritional powerhouses, I balance my diet with things that are good for me. In fact, the bulk of my diet is composed of nutritious foods that sustain me for the long haul; that fuel my brain, my muscles, and my nervous system; and that help me stay healthy and prevent disease. I've learned that I feel better when I eat more foods that are good for me than those that are bad for me, and that eating *regular*, balanced meals throughout the day feels good. I've found the key benefits of consistently eating well: I have more energy and a better disposition. My diet actually allows me to enjoy life more, and it helps me be more productive professionally.

When *Good Morning America* called me to be on air (they often ask me to appear on various nutrition segments, with topics ranging from pizzas to sports bars, heart health to food myths), they told me they were going to have on the show a woman named Tricia Cunningham, who had lost 150 pounds and had kept it off for six years, to explain how she did it. They asked me to validate or refute her method, and in particular whether it would work for a broad audience. They wanted to be sure their viewers got an authentically healthy diet and not a false claim, and I was happy to oblige.

First, I read Tricia's background notes and her story. Hers was an easy concept to support, as I'd already been working with a similar concept in my practice: caloric distribution. Essentially this means you divide your calories more evenly throughout the day and, if you do this, even at a stable weight your body composition will be better. Many of my weight-loss clients were facing the same challenges that Tricia had when she developed the Reverse Diet. Often in my practice, I see that my clients need to rethink the way they approach meals, snacks, and food in general.

When many of my clients first came to me, they were out of touch with the reality of hunger and fullness. Very often, their eating was driven by anxiety, habit, emotion, or convenience. I started by helping clients retune in to basic body signals, reorganize food selection, and alter their approach to eating. This was all part of their journey toward feeling better. Helping clients master these skills is part of what I enjoy doing as a nutritionist and it is what the Reverse Diet will do for you.

From the moment I met Tricia, I loved her honesty and energy. Her creative way of bringing her story to life is something many can relate to. Everyone has his own story and her own truth. Figuring out what the right healthy lifestyle is for you, personally, is not something you will learn from a nutritionist. We can give you the tools, help you build the skills, and give you knowledge, but in the end you will pave your own path and define your own success. My role in this book is to continue what was started when Tricia and I first appeared on *Good Morning America*: to validate what works, expand on the science and the facts behind what makes this diet successful, and make sure this diet suits everyone, no matter what the challenges.

Tricia created the Reverse Diet from her own intuition, research, successes, and failures. That is how we all learn and grow. Tricia figured out what worked for her, and had great success with it. I believe everyone can benefit from the Reverse Diet, not least because it encourages less processed food, more whole food, and a healthy eating schedule without starvation. Also it will help people recognize and modify poor habits and negative patterns, which will have a lasting positive effect on their lives.

Tricia and I have combined her real-life experience with my years of practical work in the field with hundreds of clients (including professional athletes, top executives, actors, dancers, homemakers, factory workers, and college students), to help you find your own path to well-being and a stable, healthy weight. We all know that weight loss is only one part of the journey. The real challenge is maintaining the loss. Often, it is what we learn and can integrate into the rest of our lives that ultimately leads to success. Many diets focus only on weight loss. This plan is about giving you the skills to eat well for life, not just a few weeks or months.

So go on, get out that highlighter and snuggle up in a comfortable spot. Just move out of the kitchen, because when you read at the kitchen table you are setting yourself up to munch. Read on—the journey to a healthier lifestyle has just begun!

Introduction

The Reverse Diet plan helped Tricia lose 150 pounds, and she has kept it off for over six years. This is not a short-term diet; this is an approach to healthier eating and healthier eating patterns. Our plan is based on the adage eat like a king for breakfast, a prince for lunch, and a pauper for dinner. The logic is simple: if you are going on a long-distance trip, the first thing you do is fuel up the car, right? Then you gas it up as needed throughout the trip. You don't constantly gas it up; you do so only when needed. At the end of the day, you park the car. You're done driving for the day, so there's no need to fill up the tank until the morning. Just as you fuel up when you need it most, it makes sense to eat food when you need it most to fuel daily activities. Healthy calorie distribution can be achieved by eating normal amounts of food at certain times of the day, preventing that food from being stored as fat.

Many overweight people eat only one "real" meal a day: dinner. By the time dinner rolls around, they are starving, and very often they overeat or continue snacking and munching until bedtime. Even for people who eat three meals a day, usually dinner is their largest. In the Reverse Diet, we suggest dinner for breakfast and breakfast for dinner to help people change the way they think about meals. The Reverse Diet requires you to switch the typical portions of dinner and breakfast—so you have a larger meal in the morning and a smaller meal at night. Whether those meals are breakfast or dinner foods doesn't matter. We ask only that you eat foods from the Reverse Diet Food List (basically healthy, whole, unprocessed foods), which is on pages 32 to 34.

That's the basic premise of the Reverse Diet. In the morning, you need to eat the food that will propel you throughout the day. This is the most important meal, and it should be the largest. Consuming a lot of calories, fats, carbohydrates, and proteins at the end of the day doesn't make much sense, as your body doesn't need to fuel up before it's going to be inactive, and it won't burn off much of what you take in. In the Reverse Diet, you eat the most important and largest meal—traditionally dinner—in the morning when you most need the food. Then you eat a sensible lunch—the same size as or smaller than what you ate in the morning. In the evening you eat a meal that will satiate you but doesn't add excess calories that your body won't be able to get rid of and would otherwise turn into fat. The final meal in a Reverse Diet day is smaller than what may be typical for most people. As Tricia says, when she began eating a large breakfast and a medium-size lunch of healthy foods, she was not as hungry as she previously had been at dinner.

By switching the portions of breakfast and dinner, you will eat more sensibly. Your meal in the morning will boost your energy throughout the day. Your meal at night will be something you enjoy, and it won't stick around long while you're inactive. By eating a sensible meal at night, you'll sleep better and will have a healthy appetite in the morning. Reversing your meal sizes and eating unprocessed foods forces you to question how much you should eat at certain times of the day by changing your definitions of breakfast and dinner. Instead of being restrictive, the Reverse Diet actually expands your food choices at each meal. Eventually not only do you reverse your meals, you reverse your life for the better.

The Reverse Diet eating plan is based on good, healthy, whole foods. You might be surprised at how you don't miss the fat- and sugar-laden foods you thought you could never give up. Unlike many popular diets, the Reverse Diet is a plan that you can stick with even after you achieve your weight-loss goals, because it doesn't require giving up entire food groups like carbohydrates and loading up on others like protein. You can have your juice, carrots, and potatoes and still lose weight!

How to Use This Book

Unlike most diet plans, the Reverse Diet program is not regimented by "Week 1, 2, 3" and so on. The Reverse Diet plan is unique in a few other ways, too. For example, you can personalize a good bit of the plan to suit you. If you're ready to start the diet, you can do it as soon as you begin reading this book. There's no better time than right now!

While it makes the most sense to read this book from front to back, you can also skip ahead to certain sections when you want to. Feel free to jump to the food list on page 32 if you'd like to prepare a Reverse Diet meal immediately. After doing so, continue to read the chapters in order.

Chapter 1 will help you set your goal. Chapter 2 will give you the necessary food list and initial recommendations. After that, we'll give you some essential advice to help you stay on the plan and succeed.

Three Phases That Build toward a Healthy Life

There are three phases to the Reverse Diet. The first phase is the Reverse Diet Weight-Loss Phase. In this phase you will learn how to:

- Eat healthfully at certain times of the day with a big breakfast and a smaller dinner
- Choose whole, nutritious foods from the extensive Reverse Diet Food List
- Readjust your thought process about how you eat

- Remove emotional, environmental, and motivational obstacles to better eating

After you reach your goal weight, the Reverse Diet Bridge Phase will show you how to:

- Reintroduce high-calorie foods in small portions
- Adjust your meals and eating habits so that you can keep a balanced, healthy weight
- Transition from the weight-loss phase to the maintenance phase
- Learn how to understand your emotions and reframe negative thoughts

In the Reverse Diet Maintenance Phase you will learn how to:

- Maintain your motivation
- Set new goals in life
- Keep your healthful lifestyle for life

While we devote the most attention in this book to the first phase due to the amount of information that is needed to reverse dieting and eating habits, all the phases are important. Each phase sets you up for success. Although you lose the weight in the initial phase, you concentrate on keeping the weight off in the other two phases in order to achieve a balanced weight for life. Many dieters agree that keeping weight off is the biggest challenge. Each phase is a cornerstone to escape bad eating and weight-gain cycles for good.

Throughout all three phases, this book will walk you through the challenges. The Reverse Diet plan will provide tips on surviving day to day, getting back on the wagon after slip-ups, and maintaining your success. Tricia shares her recipes, including many family favorites adapted for the Reverse Diet. The book is filled with Tricia's and Heidi's secrets for navigating any social occasion and forestalling even the worst temptation through planning. Step-by-step, we'll help you overcome your bad habits and develop good ones. You'll learn how to identify harmful, impossible ideals for weight loss you may encounter throughout your life, and how to develop manageable, healthy goals that reflect your personal truth and that will serve you best in your new lifestyle.

Across North America, people are joining the Reverse Diet way of life. With 65 percent of Americans overweight, people are looking for a working solution. Not only has this program helped our clients overcome lifelong weight issues, but many have overcome life-threatening weight issues and added years to their lives. Congratulations for picking up this book and taking the beginning steps to reverse your life!

The Reverse Diet Weight-Loss Phase

1

What Is the Reverse Diet?

I saw Tricia and Heidi on Good Morning America *and started on the diet immediately. I started at 235 pounds and in one year I have lost 85 pounds! I love eating this new way, with one big meal in the morning and smaller meals throughout the day. Now I look forward to morning meals as a time to really enjoy good food. I know I still have a little weight left to lose, but I'm happy with my results now. After this long on the diet, I'm good at maintaining. I can stay at a particular weight for as long as I want or continue on down the scale. I'm in control of how much I lose and when. I can stay on the Reverse Diet anywhere I go.*
—Becky, a successful Reverse Dieter

Welcome to the Reverse Diet. This program is not just about losing weight, it is about reframing your approach to eating. One of the first things to do as you begin the Reverse Diet is to set a goal that is achievable and that can continue to motivate you toward a healthier lifestyle. We believe setting goals is good to do before you begin the program because goals can help keep you on track and focused. In this chapter we'll go over some distinctions between healthy and unrealistic goals. At the end of the chapter, you can choose the goals you'll be working toward throughout the plan—the first step toward reversing your body and your life!

Moving toward a Reverse Lifestyle

Tricia says that no one wakes up, looks in the mirror, and says, "I want to gain a hundred and fifty pounds." Tricia never deliberately decided to gain that much weight. But, importantly, she did have to deliberately decide to lose it. You may not have decided to gain that extra 10, 50, or 100 pounds, but you realize as you examine yourself in the mirror that that is exactly what you've done. As Tricia often says to her fellow Reverse Dieters, "If you can gain the weight, you can lose the weight." Now by reading this book, you're deciding to lose that weight. With the Reverse Diet, you can make the same decision that Tricia made and take the steps toward losing weight and gaining your confidence and better quality of life.

Most likely, you were driven to start this plan because you have a glimmer of hope that you can have a different relationship with food and your body. A voice inside you may be saying, "Yes, I will finally make that change toward a healthier lifestyle." Listen closely, because that little voice can become the big voice you hear every day. With this plan, you will find the power to reverse your life. You will begin to understand that you can feel full and satisfied, and you can listen to your body signals so that you eat regular-size meals—and as you do so, you can lose weight.

Take a look at the following list and see if any of these apply to you:

- Do your clothes not fit right because of your weight?
- Is your clothes size moving up?
- Are you afraid to get on the scale?
- Do you have an upcoming event that you want to lose weight for (a wedding, a reunion, or a cruise)?
- Do you have extra post-pregnancy weight to lose?
- Have you ever been unable to see the stairs because of your belly?

- Have you ever felt embarrassed when someone saw how much you had on your plate?
- Do you get out of breath after a quick walk across the parking lot?
- Do you weight cycle (yo-yo diet, gain and lose weight each week or month)?
- Do you diet by day and overeat by night?
- Do you snack instead of eating real meals?
- When mealtime comes, are you completely unprepared—you don't know what you'll be eating, but you are starving?
- Do you eat fast food more than three times a week?
- Do you make unrealistic promises to yourself about food, such as "I'm never going to overeat again"?
- Have you ever felt yourself longing for a time in the past when you looked better, felt better, and had more energy?
- Has your doctor told you to change your diet due to high cholesterol, high blood pressure, or other health problems?
- Has your love life suffered from what you perceive to be a weight problem?
- Have you become reclusive due to your weight?
- Do you often feel lonely and blame it on your weight?

If you identified with several of these questions, the Reverse Diet is for you. Whether you want to lose 5 or 100 pounds, the change on the scale will be just one of the profound things that will happen once you lose the weight. Just as important will be what happens to your self-image, your body, your mood, your energy, and your confidence.

Reverse Diet Benefits

Once you learn to take the steps toward reversing your habits, you will see results. Some of the changes you'll begin to notice include:

- More energy. Tricia and many of her clients find they don't even need caffeine to start the day! As your metabolism soars, so do you.

- Visits to the scale will be rewarding rather than depressing.
- Improved body image. Your clothes will fit, you'll enjoy picking out what to wear, and you won't dread photo time.
- You will discover that confidence is about you and not your body, and you will come to terms with any lingering body-image issues you might have.
- You will have fewer health setbacks or issues like high blood pressure, high triglycerides, blood sugar imbalance, high cholesterol, glucose tolerance/intolerance, heart disease risk, risk of stroke, Alzheimer's, and macular degeneration.
- You will feel less stress. A healthier lifestyle reduces both physical and mental stress.
- You will enjoy better moods.

The Reverse Diet plan doesn't require the intensive consumption of certain foods that other diets do. By reversing the habits you've been taught all your life, you may find you have been starving yourself at the wrong parts of the day and filling your stomach during the time of day you need food the least—at dinner (and after dinner). Now, instead of looking forward all day long to a large meal at dinner, you'll be eating satisfying, full meals throughout the day. When you learn to look at meals differently, your body will respond with a higher metabolism and increased energy. Sugar and salt cravings will be more manageable. You will begin to see emotional eating for what it truly is: a habit. As your habits reverse, so will your past failures at dieting.

Realistic Weight versus Your Idealistic Weight: Setting Goals

When her clients begin a new diet plan, Heidi often tries to help them distinguish between *realistic* and *idealistic* weight goals. She has found that if they strive to meet realistic goals, they have a higher rate of success.

Body image or body satisfaction and the amount you weigh are two different things. The Reverse Diet plan encourages the emphasis to be put on positive body image rather than a specific amount to weigh.

Take a moment to think about what you idealistically would like to weigh. How would you like your body to look? How far from reality or possibility is that image? Most of us have an idealistic weight goal. Weight loss won't change our height, for example, or our basic features. We are taught by the popular media to want something that many of us will never have, a so-called perfect body. How often do you disparage a particular feature of yours? Do you look specifically for fat rolls because in our culture you are *ideally* supposed to have none? You might so constantly be asking yourself what is wrong with your body instead of what is right that it is no wonder you have distanced yourself from your body. So often, our thoughts and our impressions about what is good and what is bad are based on unrealistic aesthetics instead of realistic health.

Many people begin programs by choosing the specific number of pounds they would like to lose. Examine what your ideals are and what exactly is motivating you before you seek that goal weight.

Are you influenced by realistic standards? The media and Hollywood motivate us to desire bodies that many of us will never have. Perhaps you don't have the correct build for a body like Jennifer Aniston's or you don't have the time or energy to devote to exercise and a perfect diet. Remember, *perfect* is different from *healthy*. This is true for diets and for people. With idealistic goals, no matter how much we try, we rarely will reach them no matter what we sacrifice to get there. Making the sacrifices required to reach these goals takes away from other things we value in our lives. You may rarely reach an idealistic weight goal or may sustain it for only short periods of time, in comparison with getting to a stable weight that is healthy for the rest of your life.

What Goals Do You Strive For?

Take a moment to look over the following list and figure out what unexamined, unrealistic ideals you have been harboring. Perhaps you've always wanted certain things but have never actually examined your goals. Do you hope to accomplish these things?

If you find the right diet plan and lose weight, you will:

- Lose 10 pounds every week for six months
- Have no stretch marks
- Have no sagging skin
- Have no love handles
- Have no rolls of fat or jiggling body parts
- Look the way you did before puberty
- Look the way you did the day of your wedding
- Look like (insert name of supermodel or actor of choice)
- Have a perfect life (be smarter, more outgoing, financially successful)
- Never overeat
- Look fifteen years younger
- Go from a size 14 to a size 2
- Get the perfect man or woman
- Be taller, have longer legs, or have a different body altogether

How many of these things haunt you and produce more and more guilt and feelings of inadequacy and failure when you find you cannot live up to them? Do you feel you will be able to fulfill these expectations for the rest of your life without dramatic sacrifices or misery? How many goals do you think you can achieve long-term? How many are about more than just what you weigh on the scale?

These ideals aren't necessarily impossible, but you should evaluate what you really think you can do and feel good about without sacrificing the quality of the rest of your life. Remember, success and health may entail some sacrifice. Not sacrificing in order to reach your goal is a myth. Getting what you want by putting very little to no effort forth is a myth. What matters is when and where you put the effort. The Reverse Diet plan will help you figure out where your effort will pay off and where it won't.

Let's Get Reverse Real

A realistic weight is one you can achieve by eating healthfully, moderately, and regularly. Realistic goals are goals that concentrate on an inside-out healthy lifestyle. Better feelings about yourself and better eating habits equal a better quality of life. No harsh standards or negativity go along with realistic goals. Realistic goals include the possibility of falling off the wagon and not beating yourself up for it. These goals focus on your being healthy at age fifty-five rather than wearing a size 5 at age thirty. That doesn't mean you can't look great at any age. Looking healthy, trim, and fit is different from looking skinny.

What the Reverse Diet Can Do for You

If you commit to the Reverse Diet plan, you will:

- Have better eating habits you can keep throughout life
- Develop more awareness about how to eat well easily
- Have long-term results and a healthy stabilized weight
- Gain the satisfaction of setting *and* achieving goals
- Feel comfortable in your clothes
- Gain more confidence
- Have a healthier, more active lifestyle
- Have more energy throughout the day
- Enjoy food without denying yourself or sacrificing full meals
- Lose fat and not muscle
- Leave behind your negative body images
- Quiet the critical voices in your head about your weight and appearance
- Have less guilt about your appearance and what you eat regularly
- Be able to walk up the stairs without losing your breath
- Live a longer, fuller life so that you can have fun and play with your grandchildren one day

How many of these goals produce a positive emotion? Are these benefits or goals you would like to keep throughout your life? Read on to find out what action steps will help you achieve them. And when you become realistic and healthy, it will become a lot easier to lose weight.

Tricia found when she was able to maintain 130 pounds, she enjoyed her lifestyle more than when she attempted to stay at 125. At 5'8", 125 felt too skinny, and it demanded that she make sacrifices that interrupted her quality of life. At 130, she is able to enjoy an energetic lifestyle without the stress of thinking that she won't reach a nearly impossible weight goal. When Tricia finally decided she just wanted to be healthy and to lead an active, longer life with her family, she began to push aside ideal weight goals and work toward realistic weight goals. That was when her long-term success began.

Your Reverse Diet Journal

It's important that you keep a journal as you follow the Reverse Diet plan. Find what works for you. It can be a notebook, a blank book, or a folder on your computer or on your personal data assistant. It's up to you. Your journal is a very special tool in the Reverse Diet plan. You will use it every day.

How Do You Cut Your Pie?

If you are overweight or have been, you know that it can cut into the quality of your life by consuming inordinate amounts of brain space and time thinking about food, feeling guilty about eating, and obsessing about what you look like. Tricia's life was dominated by her weight issues before she developed the Reverse Diet. All of us want to feel good in our clothes and be proud of our figures, but we should also focus on parts of our lives other than when we're going to have a brownie sundae, or if we've had the brownie sundae, how bad we feel because we had it. Many of our clients obsess over what they ate and what they weigh so often that ultimately they are wasting valuable energy when they could be directing it toward reversing their lives. They spend time feeling bad about what they ate, rather than dealing with the emotion that drove them to overeat or to eat something unhealthy.

What are the different elements that make up your daily life now? The goal is to broaden your life beyond food in meaningful ways. Think of these things as slices of a pie. If you're like most people, the sections of your pie are:

Work

Family

Intellectual activity

Health/wellness/
   physical issues/weight

Emotional concerns

Spiritual concerns

Cultural concerns

Social concerns

How I look (weight)

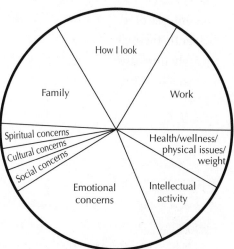

With this in mind, it's important to evaluate how much of your life will be focused on how you look and what you weigh. Of course it's great to have pride in how you look, but that is different from having your day ruined by bad hair or a shift on the scale. Do you have hobbies or specific areas you want to add to this pie? The piece of the pie that is focused on health and weight supports the other parts of your life. If you give all areas of your life more attention, you will find yourself more satisfied.

REVERSE DIET EXERCISE

Draw Your Life Pie

Take a moment to draw your own pie in your journal. Design the pie so it reflects how much emphasis you currently give specific areas of your life. Do you work all the time and have little time for your family? Do you give your looks little thought? If this is the case, work should have a large slice and the other areas should have smaller slices. We can't tell you how it should be; everyone's pie will look different. Ask yourself what reflects your values and priorities.

Now draw another circle and design how you would realistically like your pie to look. If you think you work too much, make the work slice a bit smaller than in the first pie, and draw the family and looks slices a little larger. How can you reach your personal goals? How much of your pie is taken up by health or weight issues?

Your Goal Weight

Your personal objectives may be very different from other people's personal objectives. Every person has a different body, a different build, and different expectations. The Reverse Diet is designed so you can personalize it to your own tastes, habits, and goals.

Keep your realistic goal weight and broader goals in mind as you continue on the Reverse Diet. With your realistic goals in mind, choose a goal weight or weight range before you start the program. Your waist will shrink as your confidence increases.

REVERSE DIET EXERCISE

Write Down Your Goal

Take a moment to write down at the front of your journal one or more personal, realistic goals. Pick a goal that is achievable, like many of the realistic goals listed previously in this chapter. It might be something like "Freedom from weight cycling" or "Achieve a balanced, healthy weight I can maintain for life." If you want to select a weight, find a range instead. Instead of picking a goal weight of 140 pounds, for example, make it a range from 140 to 145. This will help put less emphasis on a specific number and more on the general state of health you will be in when you reach that range.

Remember, we're talking about not only how great it will feel when you reach your goal but what it will take to get there. Next, we'll discuss developing the skills you need to achieve your goals. Put your realistic goal aside so that you can come back and refer to it throughout the Reverse Diet program.

Take a picture of yourself, if you like. It can be helpful at certain parts of the plan to look back at your "before" picture. You're going to feel fantastic when you see how far you've come.

Form Better Habits

As you work toward your goal weight range, remember that you should focus on the process and action steps you're taking to get there rather than the actual number of pounds you hope to weigh. Throughout the book we will help you build the skills you need and help you identify the actions you can take to achieve your goals. It takes action to reach a goal. When you focus on the process of the Reverse Diet—when you eat, what you eat, how you eat, and why you eat—you will be building a foundation of new habits that will support a more stable, healthy weight. If you simply have blinders on and concentrate on the goal weight you hope to achieve, once you reach that weight, you may have difficulty staying there, because you haven't been entirely focused on the new process of healthy living. Achieving your goal weight range is something that happens as you learn the process and action steps toward a healthy lifestyle. Change your habits and form better ones, and weight loss will follow.

Your Reverse Diet Moment

Almost everyone has a Reverse Diet moment—when they realize that they have to make a change for the better. Tricia had hers, and it was the catalyst for a new life for both her and her family.

Tricia was a chronic yo-yo dieter; there had been many, many times when she decided to lose weight and would do it. Eventually, though, other things would take over her weight-loss goal and she would gain the weight back. Although she would try to succeed, she encountered many obstacles. Sometimes her schedule at work would become overwhelming or the kids didn't want to eat healthy foods, or she told herself, "I just don't have the stamina to eat healthy."

Now that she has had her Reverse Diet moment, she says, "There is not one excuse you can throw at me that cannot be overcome. I have been there and done it all."

What will your Reverse Diet moment be? Maybe it has happened. Perhaps learning about someone like Tricia who has lost that much weight and kept if off is your inspiration. Perhaps picking up this book and beginning this plan is preparing you for your moment. You must ask yourself, are you ready for *your* moment? There is no better time than right now.

REVERSE DIET EXERCISE

Become Aware of Your Reverse Potential

Take the time today to stand in front of the mirror. What are the first few things you see? What are the thoughts you have about your body? Record in your journal everything you see and what you feel. Take note if you experience mostly negative thoughts. Ask yourself if you are ready to love and embrace the person in the mirror. This is your chance to reverse things and begin to appreciate your body and yourself. Work on becoming aware of negative, damaging thoughts that could potentially sabotage your goals to remake your life and your body.

Throughout the Reverse Diet plan you'll work on reframing your thoughts so that much of the way you feel toward your body is positive rather than negative. For example, instead of saying, "I have fat thighs or rolls of fat on my belly," try "I have kind eyes. My hands are beautiful. My legs are strong." It's okay to be realistic—if you are overweight, it's okay to acknowledge that—but that is not who you are, and it is not the only thing about your physical person that matters. Eventually you will look back over what you have recorded in your journal so you can begin to notice changes in your thought processes and your body. Now let's grab that Reverse Diet moment and turn the page toward a new life!

REVERSE DIET EXERCISE

Shed Idealistic Images

Stop a few times today and notice—are you recycling old negative thoughts about your body image? Listen closely, because these thoughts are not going to help you reverse your life. The more you become aware of them, the less damage they can do.

Begin to take notice of the unrealistic, idealistic body image goals that are being pushed on you every day. Do you subscribe to a certain magazine that features airbrushed models? Do you watch MTV or soap operas and wonder why you don't look like a pop star? Do you work with someone who is petite and constantly feel inadequate around her? Every time you see one of these idealistic body goals pushed at you, counter it with a positive thought and remember your personal, realistic goal with a smile.

2

The Reverse Diet Food List and Reverse Diet Basics

The Reverse Diet is the first diet I have ever been on where I feel completely in control of what I eat. I also feel energized throughout the day. My motivation comes from knowing that I'm eating healthy, and of course, the results on the scale! I have lost 25 pounds, down from 170 pounds, on the Reverse Diet so far. Tricia's theory about eating your largest meal in the morning makes complete sense and it's something we should all do every day. It's truly the best diet I have ever followed, and I hope more and more people learn about this amazing diet so they can know what it feels like to be at a healthy weight and finally feel in control of what they eat.

—Marissa, a successful Reverse Dieter

Flip-Flop Your Day to Keep the Weight Away

Now that you have your realistic weight goal, it will be helpful to become familiar with a few important tools on the plan. In this chapter, you'll get the basics on how to begin the diet so that you can reach your goal, and you'll learn about some of the science behind why it works.

As you know by now, the concept is simple: eat your dinner for breakfast and your breakfast for dinner. The diet is simple: just eat a well-balanced menu of unrefined and healthier food choices. That is why so many people are so successful at it. You don't have to eat actual breakfast foods for dinner and actual dinner foods for breakfast throughout the whole diet if you don't want to, but it's a good way to start just so you get used to eating a more well-rounded morning meal with protein and unrefined carbohydrates in place of pastries, breakfast breads, doughnuts, and breakfast meats like sausage. This diet gives you a greater range of selections than just typical breakfast foods. Try it—you'll be used to it before you know it.

Whatever you do, do not skip breakfast. Skipping breakfast altogether is one of the biggest ways to sabotage your diet and your body's metabolism. An important element of the plan is to reverse your meal sizes, times, and content to better distribute your calories throughout the day. In your daily menu we recommend consuming around one-third of your calories when you first wake for the day, then have a medium-size meal at lunch, your smallest meal at dinner, and *planned* healthy snacks in between meals as needed. Eat like a king in the morning, a prince at lunch, and a pauper at dinner.

Although the plan encourages larger meals in the beginning of the day and snacks when necessary, the program does not allow for the unlimited consumption of foods. Instead, you should use the Reverse Diet Food List to be creative and personalize your plan by eating the foods on the list that you enjoy in appropriate portions.

If you have not already begun the plan, start it today by eating a light dinner early in the evening and your larger meal of the day tomorrow morning. Go ahead and plan your first Reverse Diet breakfast with the Reverse Diet Food List on pages 32 to 34. If you are not used to eating a large breakfast or any breakfast, it may feel strange at first, but don't worry, you will soon wake up craving a well-rounded meal. Successful Reverse Dieters have found that their bodies adjust well to the new routine.

The Reverse Diet Food List
(Weight-Loss Phase)

Following is a sample list of the foods Tricia ate during the first phase of the Reverse Diet. (Note that "moderation/sparingly" qualify as no more than three times per week in a mindful portion.) She stuck to whole, natural foods, and cut down on sugar, salt, and processed foods. As you put together your meals, you will learn how to make the Reverse Diet Food List work for you. Pretty soon, you'll know what's on the Reverse Diet Food List without having to refer to it. Check out www.thereversedietsolution.com for Heidi's and Tricia's favorite brands.

Vegetables

All (including carrots, potatoes, and corn), fresh and frozen, with no added butter or salt

Grains

All whole grain flours

Whole grain bread sparingly

Brown rice (including instant brown rice)

Long grain wild rice

Healthy, whole grain cereals

Rolled oats/oatmeal

Barley

Grits, no salt

Bulgar

Wheat bran

Wheat germ

Matzo

Rice or popcorn cakes, unseasoned

Popcorn

Unsalted whole grain crackers (whole wheat melba toast and others)

Low-sodium tortilla shells

No-sodium/baked tortilla chips

Whole wheat/whole grain pita bread, English muffin

Millet

Spelt

Tapioca flour

Soy flour

Rice flour

Corn meal, no salt

Whole wheat pasta ($\frac{1}{2}$ to 1 cup, cooked, at a time and no more than 3 times per week at first)

Fruits/Juices

All whole fruit, fresh or frozen (no sugar added)

Unsweetened 100% cranberry juice

Orange juice

No-sugar-added prune juice

Pomegranate juice

Dairy

Light soy milk

Light soy yogurt

Fat-free plain yogurt

Ultra-fat-free (nonfat) or skim milk (in moderation)

Meats/Proteins

All chicken/turkey, skinless

Eggs

All types of fish unprepared or unbreaded (including low-sodium tuna in a can packed in water)

Fat-free cottage cheese

Low-fat white cheese (low-sodium content)

Low-fat ricotta cheese

Parmesan cheese

Lean beef—sirloin, round, flank

Tofu, firm or extra-firm

Tempeh

FATS
Nuts

Dry, unsalted nuts and seeds (all in limited portions due to fat content—⅓ cup at a time)

Nut or seed butter (sparingly) including sugar-free almond butter and peanut butter

Oils

Sesame seed oil

Extra-virgin olive oil

Canola oil

Olive oil-based salad dressings (no more than 2 teaspoons at a time or approximately 10 grams of fat)

Other

Avocadoes

Unsalted butter (no more than 2 teaspoons at a time or approximately 10 grams of fat)

Low-fat margarine or butter substitute

Low-fat or no-fat mayo (sparingly)

Fat-free sour cream (could be under condiments)

Fat-free cream cheese (watch sodium; could be under condiments)

Seasonings

All (except salt) with no added salt or sugar

Condiments (use sparingly)

Hot sauce

Fat-free salad dressing (any kind with less than 350 milligrams of sodium per serving) or low-fat dressing with less than 3 grams of fat per serving; these tend to have less sugar in them

Horseradish

Low-sodium soy sauce

Ketchup

Mustard

Red wine vinegar

Apple cider vinegar

Balsamic vinegar

Rice vinegar

Honey (very sparingly)

Desserts/Snacks (sparingly)

Sugar-free/fat-free gelatins and puddings

Fat-free/sugar-free popsicles

Whipped cream, only light or fat-free/sugar-free

Fat-free/sugar-free ice cream with no higher than 90 milligrams of sodium

Fat-free frozen yogurt

These Items Should Not Be Eaten during Weight Loss

Canned or jarred vegetables, or frozen vegetables with added butter, salt, or sauce

Frozen fruits with added sugar

Ham smoked with added salt and sugar

Non–whole grain, processed crackers

Sugary cereals

Peanut butter with sugar and salt added

Jelly

Canned or jarred/boxed gravies, sauces, fruits, veggies, or meats (except low-sodium tuna, sardines, clams, oysters)

Yellow cheeses

Boxed rice/pasta dinners

Hot dogs

Kielbasa

Fried foods

Fast foods

Turn to this list when you're in doubt about any type food you're about to eat. If you're not sure if it's on the list, take a look and see. The bulk of this list is made up of unpackaged, unprocessed healthy whole foods. They are easy to find, and there are plenty of different ways to prepare them. See the recipes in chapter 9 for Tricia's favorite Reverse Diet foods.

A note to vegetarians or vegans: The Reverse Diet is perfectly fine for you, too! You may need to add more soy, beans, nuts, and seeds to consume adequate protein; load up on vegetables; and round out your meal plan with grains and fruits. See your health care provider to ensure you are getting all the vitamins and minerals you need such as calcium and B_{12}.

REVERSE DIET EXERCISE

Determine Your Trigger Foods

Take a moment to make a short list of your trigger foods in your journal. Do you have a particular food that you regularly overeat? If so, take note and be aware that you must be very careful of that food during the weight-loss phase of the Reverse Diet plan.

Now that you've recorded your trigger foods, take another look at the Reverse Diet Food List. How many of your trigger foods are on the Reverse Diet list? If there are several on the list— great! When you eat those foods, you'll just have to focus on timing and portion size. If there are few or none of your personal trigger foods on the list, you'll have to be especially careful and learn how to greatly cut down on them. If they are not on the list, it may be helpful to try to eliminate them from your diet for the time being.

Keep the Reverse Diet Food List in an accessible place. Some of our clients keep a copy in the kitchen, others in their planners or purses. Figure out where you will most likely need it when you get ready to make your shopping list.

Eventually and inevitably, there will be times when you will give in to your cravings or old overeating habits. The big difference is noticing and regulating your cravings. One of Tricia's favorite cravings is for nachos. She does one of two things: she allows herself to have them every once in a while in a controlled portion size or she prepares them with much healthier ingredients than are in your typical nachos (baked chips, black beans, vegetables, and low-fat white or nacho cheese). You have the same option on this plan—you will learn how to tweak almost any recipe to make the selection of ingredients and preparation better for you.

Tricia's Reverse Diet Days

Here are some sample menus of typical days for Tricia when she first began the Reverse Diet. Most of these recipes can be found in the Reverse Diet recipe chapter. This will give you an example of the type of meals and portion sizes you can begin with. We include two full weeks of meal plans in the next chapter. Enjoy!

Day 1

Breakfast

　　1 cup of cooked whole wheat pasta

　　10 medium shrimp, lightly sautéed

Snack

　　2 plums with 4 ounces of skim milk

Lunch

　　Grilled chicken breast on a bed of mixed greens with olive oil dressing, and served with 2 slices of tomato

Snack

　　An apple with 2 ounces of cubed part-skim mozzarella cheese

Dinner

　　2 hard-boiled eggs and tofu served with a salad of tomato, corn, and cucumber

Day 2

Breakfast

　　A two-egg omelet mixed with 2 cups of a mix of spinach, cauliflower, broccoli, and garlic

Snack

　　½ cup of cereal mixed with 4 ounces of skim milk and 10 walnuts

Lunch

　　Stuffed tomato: 1 large tomato with the top cut off, the insides spooned into a bowl containing a can of tuna, tofu, celery, onions, and spices; the ingredients are mixed and stuffed in the tomato. The tomato is served on a bed of lettuce.

Snack

1 cup of blueberries with 1 cup of low-fat plain yogurt

Dinner

1½ cups of uncooked oatmeal and shredded wheat with 4 ounces of orange juice

1 cup of green beans and tofu

As you can see, you eat real food at each meal, distributing your calories throughout the day. You can always mix up having breakfast foods at breakfast or dinner and lunch foods at breakfast. Do what's comfortable for you.

Reversing What and When

Some diets tell you to have a particular combination of foods, exclude carbohydrates, eat fruit only at certain times of the day, and so on. The Reverse Diet doesn't have those types of complications. Yes, everyone should have a certain amount of veggies, protein, and starchy carbohydrates, but you don't have to make this the ultimate focus of every meal.

That said, it's helpful to use some old-fashioned common sense about the food groups when you choose what makes up each meal. There are six food groups. Become aware of the food groups you're eating from. Try to eat at least one serving from two or three groups at each meal. For example, if you eat all dairy and carbohydrates in the morning, work on having a protein and vegetables at lunch and then vegetables and fruits in the evening. Better yet, attempt to distribute your groups evenly each day. When you are deciding what to have for your next meal, consider what you had the meal before. You don't want to have only the same food groups; you want to balance your nutrition intake by hitting all of them.

The Six Food Groups

Vegetables: Vary your vegetables; get your greens daily and orange vegetables at least every other day.

Fruits: Choose at least one vitamin C–rich fruit a day.

Milk and yogurt: Make sure you get your calcium through low-fat dairy.

Grains: Bread, cereal, rice, and pasta; at least three whole grains a day.

Proteins: Meat, poultry, fish, dry beans, eggs, and cheese; protein helps you feel full–go lean.

Fats: Oils and sweets; your body needs healthy fats (unsaturated, monounsaturated fats) daily, but sweets are discretionary calories and *if* included, should be limited to 10 to 15 percent of total calories each day.

For example, in a 1,500-calorie diet, you should have 3 whole grains, 3 starches, 3 vegetables, 2 fruits, 3 dairies, another 8-ounce serving of protein, and 30 to 40 grams of fat. (See appendix C.) Heidi had one client, Norman, who made a great many adjustments in his life. He had begun eating larger breakfasts, medium-size lunches, and smaller dinners. After looking at his food journal, though, Heidi noticed that he ate too much starch at each meal and not enough vegetables. For example, one morning he had a turkey sandwich with a pasta salad. Although he had a little bit of protein, for the most part, most of his meal was starch. While it was low-fat, only two of the food groups were represented. Heidi advised Norman to try a turkey sandwich and a salad or fruit next time and to keep the different food groups in mind when he chose his meals.

When you choose your meals, make sure you're eating foods from the Reverse Diet Food List in reasonable portions at the times of day your body needs them the most. We will discuss portions in detail in chapter 4. Our emphasis is on when you eat, what you eat, and how much you eat. This will help you become more aware of when your body needs food rather than listening to regimented restrictions on food combinations or calorie counting. Those can take away from your attention to your body. Eventually you will work toward balancing your portions, but don't make this your central focus in the beginning. Until you get the hang of eating in the Reverse Diet way, tune in to your body and experiment with different types of meals. Listen to what your body wants to eat from our food list.

Sometimes you may want a steak, another time eggs or pasta, or you might crave a particular texture or taste—crunchy, chewy, creamy, spicy, or tangy. Consider what will ultimately nourish you, not just satisfy an immediate impulse.

One Reverse Dieter said, "I used to eat too much of one food regularly. Maybe it was bread, or too much protein, but now I realize I'm satisfied when I round off my meals with vegetables and a sensible portion of protein."

Dinner Foods at Breakfast Time

As we've said, you don't necessarily need to eat dinner foods at breakfast time, but it does expand your choices. You can mix it up. Omelets are perfectly fine for breakfast, just make sure they are Reverse Diet portions (more about that later). Get creative or stay with what you like, as long as it's healthy. Either way, there are a lot of recipes to choose from in the recipe chapter. Whether it's a typical "dinner meal" with protein and veggies or a vegetable omelet, find foods you like and combinations that work for you. Just make sure they are on the Reverse Diet Food List.

If you're in the habit of skipping breakfast or having a delayed breakfast or lunch, reteach your metabolism to crave that morning meal. By making sure that you eat *no later than one hour after you wake up,* you are jump-starting your metabolism immediately. If you don't eat soon after you wake up, your body doesn't have fuel to burn when you start your day. When you are sleeping, you are also fasting for an average of about eight hours in addition to the time since your last meal before bedtime, so it's essential to break this fast. Eating in the morning gives you a boost. People who skip breakfast often catch up on their energy requirements later in the day, yet they're unlikely to get all the vitamins and minerals that a simple breakfast can provide. And people who miss breakfast often snack by midmorning on foods that are high in sugar or fat. One study showed that those who typically skip breakfast and eat only at lunch did more poorly on memory tests and were tired by noon only four hours after they awoke.

Calorie Distribution

When Tricia began the diet, she simply tried to eat healthful meals with foods she knew were better than much of the junk food she typically ate. She stumbled onto the fact that if she ate a well-rounded meal for breakfast, a medium one for lunch, and a small one for dinner, she would lose weight. As Tricia lost more and more weight on the Reverse Diet, she soon came to realize why it was working. She had learned how to distribute her calories throughout the day.

In order to adjust your mind-set to this new calorie distribution, it's helpful to think about your body as if it were a car. If you are about to take a long-distance trip, one of the first things you do is to fill up the tank so you do not have to keep stopping along the way. You will top off your tank when necessary. When you have reached your final destination, the last thing you want to do is run around looking for a gas station to fill up a tank that is just going to sit in a parking lot all night. Many people do the opposite to their bodies: at the beginning of the day, they eat a small meal, and at the end of the day, they eat a large one—right when they need the food the least, before bed. In essence, these people are dieting all day and eating all night, and that doesn't make sense.

Many people who begin the Reverse Diet have the bad habit of undereating during the day and overeating at night, even after having an adequate dinner. This is what Heidi calls *residual hunger*.

They "refrigerator surf," nibbling and eating throughout the evening until going to bed. This interferes with sleep and over a period of time creates a negative eating cycle. For most of us, sleeping on a full stomach does not provide a good night's sleep. Lack of sleep is an independent contributor to weight gain; cortisol levels increase when you don't get adequate sleep, and cortisol encourages belly fat. Higher cortisol levels can also interfere with our appetite regulatory hormones, so it's harder to know when you're really hungry.

One reason this constant eating occurs at night is that it is when people find themselves tired, and this puts them at higher risk for overeating. Fatigue makes it harder to resist bad habits. When overeating occurs at night, it can make people reluctant to eat a substantial breakfast in the morning or to wake earlier to allow time for breakfast.

How do you escape the after-dark residual hunger? Eat more earlier in the day, eat less at night, and go to sleep before you are exhausted. Get a better night's sleep, and you'll be less vulnerable to late-night eating. In the morning, have a well-rounded breakfast that is filling and nutritious.

Think of your body as a fuel-burning machine. Give it an appropriate meal right before the day begins and a smaller meal when it ends. You'll find that instead of storing that fuel as fat, you'll burn it off all day long. Keep this in mind as you start the diet and as you train your body to burn fuel instead of storing it.

The Hunger Scale

After a week or two on the Reverse Diet, you'll begin to find that you can control your portions and be able to tune in to your hunger signals in a way that works for you. Everyone has unique impulses. In order to determine your own way of implementing the Reverse Diet plan, you must learn to tell the difference between your old eating habits and the messages your body sends you when it needs certain things. When you listen to when your body wants to eat but you do not immediately revert to the old habit of eating a giant portion size, you will be able to limit your portions. It's also easier to avoid huge portions if you listen to when your body is hungry rather than waiting until it's starving, which can drive you to binge. For example, when you think, "I'm a little hungry, I'd like a snack," listen! Don't put it off because you think you can and you are trying to save calories, or because you think that somehow it is healthier to avoid a snack. Sometimes, by eating a snack you are better able to control portion size in your meals. Just make the snack a healthy one.

Snacking can help you avoid this scenario: "I'm starving. I could eat a horse! I'm going to the all-you-can-eat buffet to pig out!" That's an old habit talking, not your body. If your body is starving, give it reasonable nourishment and then stop when you are full. Experiment with a small portion first to see if it satisfies.

On a scale of 1 to 10 (1 being starving and 10 being stuffed) how hungry are you when you begin to eat? How full are you when you stop eating? If you have only considered this after the fact, then it is time to tune in to the Hunger Scale.

The Hunger Scale is a tool you can use to help reconnect to your body's signals, to know when you are physiologically hungry instead of emotionally, psychologically, or impulsively hungry. Recognizing true hunger cues will help you be more mindful about when to eat and how much to eat. It will help you recognize when to stop eating before that "I am stuffed" feeling comes over you. It helps you to learn appropriate portion sizes based on your needs, not on what a restaurant has determined is a good value.

Here is a tip: if you wait until you are starving, you are more likely to eat until you are stuffed. Eat when you are hungry, stop when you are just before full (start eating meals at around 2 or 3 on the scale, stop when around 8). Meal size should match hunger size. Slightly hungry, eat a snack; really hungry, eat a meal. When you're slightly hungry and you eat a huge meal, you're disregarding what your body is telling you. Being really hungry and trying to get by with a snack is the same thing: you are disregarding your body's signal. This is sure to backfire eventually. Eat when you are hungry, don't eat when you're not hungry, and eat a small amount when you're slightly hungry.

HUNGER SCALE

Empty				Empty		Full		Full	
1	2	3	4	5	6	7	8	9	10
Extremely hungry, unable to function	Very hungry but functioning	Hungry, with tolerable discomfort	Mildly hungry, can wait to eat	Neutral, not hungry, not full	Aware of food in stomach but still hungry	Full/ satisfied, with some room in stomach	Comfortably full	Too full, with some discomfort	Very uncomfortable, can't function

REVERSE DIET EXERCISE

Review the Hunger Scale

Take a look at the Hunger Scale diagram. It's a good idea to record a copy of this on an index card or just photocopy it and have it in an accessible place. When you are trying to decide if you should have a snack or not, mentally review where you stand on the Hunger Scale. Soon you will be able gauge it without the diagram.

Your Reverse Diet Journal

As we mentioned in chapter 1, you should keep a journal. In it, keep a food diary to record all the food you eat. Your journal will be a place for you to write about your experiences, your goals, and any events in your life you want to meditate on. Use the Reverse Diet diary template on page 45—you can choose how to duplicate it. If you have a spiral notebook, you can draw the template on each page, or you can photocopy the template and make multiple copies and put it in a folder or notebook. Some clients keep theirs on their computers or personal data assistants. If you want this on your computer, you can go to our Web site, www.reversedietsolution.com, and download the template. Whatever format works for you is what you should go with. At the bottom of this template, make sure you reserve space to add comments, thoughts, and general experiences at the end of your day.

Once you have a journal that works for you, make every effort to be honest when recording things in it. As you begin the Reverse Diet plan, it's okay to have slip-ups or overeating episodes. These occurrences will help you to learn how to avoid them in the future and perhaps even learn to recognize what caused them. It's helpful if you approach these incidents with the realistic attitude that they will happen. If after two weeks you have selectively entered only foods that represent fourteen days of perfect eating instead of entering when and how you overate, you have robbed yourself of the very purpose of your journal. The purpose is to begin to see general patterns or cycles of overeating or undereating followed by overeating, and to find out what kicks off those cycles. Note the types of foods you select and when you eat. The more obvious these patterns become, the more aware you can be so you can prevent or change them.

Success with the Reverse Diet plan depends on honesty. Be honest with yourself, and you will begin to see how you can retune in to your body.

In the food column, be specific. For example, two double-stuffed-cheese meat-lover pizza slices is a lot different from a thin crust, low-fat, cheese-veggie piece of pizza. Being specific will force you to look more closely at what you're eating and the choices you are making, along with the obvious and subtle differences between certain types of food.

Rate your hunger. Rate your hunger before and after you eat. Use the Hunger Scale with 1 as the most hungry you can feel and 10 as the least hungry. After paying attention to your hunger every time you eat, you'll begin to understand how much to eat and when. Soon you'll be able to detect whether or not you're eating when you're

FOOD AND BEVERAGE JOURNAL

Time	Food/Beverage	Mood	Activity	Rate Hunger before Eating 1 = Starving 10 = Full	Rate Fullness after Eating 1 = Starving 10 = Full	Optional
						Grains/starches Whole grains: Starches: Sweets:
						Meal/poultry/ fish/other
						Dairy
						Vegetables
						Fruits
						Fats
						Alcohol
						Water

Observations for the day (what worked, what didn't, what I feel good about, what I might try differently next time): _____

_____

_____

_____

_____

_____

actually hungry, and you'll tune in to what fills you up and what doesn't. Be on the lookout for these trends in your eating habits:

- When you wait too long to eat, you might be starving and you might overeat.
- When you eat when you're not hungry, take a good look to see what is motivating you to eat.
- When you overeat long after you're full, you're ignoring the full signal and eating until you're stuffed.

Pay attention to the feelings and messages your body sends you as these scenarios play out. Begin to recognize and honor the feeling you have; eat before you're starving and stop eating when your body tells you your stomach is 65 to 85 percent full. Take a break from eating, and then give yourself permission to eat again a bit later. If you are hungry, avoid the tendency to think, "I better eat all of this now because I may not eat later." Begin to find solutions to your own eating cycles. Your journal will help you review and problem-solve if you keep it diligently.

Rate your emotions. In the emotions category, make sure you write down what you are feeling when you eat. Are you feeling a little down or bored when you reach for those cookies? Are you angry about something when you eat a whole plate of nachos by yourself? Did something happen to make you feel elated and you are now celebrating with food? Try to get in touch with your emotions when you're eating. Tricia found that when she overate, she was very often in a poor emotional state. Sometimes she was feeling sad or bad about herself. Note if you feel guilty after you eat.

Record what you're doing. For the activity column, list whatever you have just finished or are in the middle of. For example, we have one client, Sally, who eats when she talks on the phone. She might eat a whole pint of ice cream without realizing it while she gossips with her friends. Do you eat a whole meal while cleaning up after dinner? Do you munch on what might be the equivalent of a full meal while preparing the meal for the rest of the family? Do you eat in front of the computer? Do you pig out after exercise? Throughout the Reverse

Diet plan, you should focus on what you're eating and what you're doing when you're eating. That way, you will establish more constructive and mindful eating patterns.

Take note of the time. Writing down the time when you eat will help you see other patterns. For example, a habit like eating chips every day at 4 p.m. can add up. One client thought she was eating mostly fruits and veggies for snacks, but realized when she looked at her journal she was eating chips around 4 p.m. three times a week! Also note if you are waiting too long in between meals (that is, lunch at 12 p.m., dinner at 8 p.m., and so on).

This journal is for your eyes only. Unless you want them to, no one else has to see it. It can be your private confessional and diary about when you eat and what you feel when you eat. Be regular and honest in your records. The journal will be one of your most valuable tools on the Reverse Diet plan.

Reverse Diet Tips

Here's a quick list of tips that would be good to read over at least once a week so that you familiarize yourself with key basics of the Reverse Diet. There will be more detail throughout the book about why these tips work, but for now try to stick to them in the beginning phases of the plan.

- Never skip breakfast.
- Eat a big breakfast. If you do not normally make breakfast in the morning, save tonight's dinner for tomorrow's breakfast.
- Eat when you're hungry, not when you're full. Do not overfill your tank. Your body tells you when it is full. Learn to listen.
- Give yourself permission to eat again, before the next meal, if you get hungry. It is easier to stop eating when you are 65 to 85 percent full. You don't continue eating because you will know there is another meal or snack around the corner.

- When you take a deep breath while eating, it is past time to stop!
- Limit servings of whole wheat pasta and brown rice to three or four times a week and don't eat them on the same day.
- Limit your salt intake to 2,300 milligrams of sodium per day. Most Americans eat an average of 10,000 milligrams per day. Start looking at food labels for sodium content.
- Stay away from prepackaged meals. They're loaded with salt and additives.
- Remember, include what you *really* eat in your journal. No one expects you to be perfect all of the time. Try to include all of the details you can remember. This will help you begin to learn what your high-risk times are so you can plan for them and be prepared.
- When you keep your journal, look back and notice patterns, timing, portion trends, high-risk times, trigger foods, foods or meals that satiate, emotional responses, and what works for you and what doesn't.
- When you are in the grocery store, buy whole foods, not processed foods. Look for the least processed foods you can find.
- As you choose your meals throughout the day, keep calorie distribution in mind. Try to get a majority of your calories in the morning and at lunch. By two-thirds of the way through your day, two-thirds of your daily food should be consumed. That way, you won't need to eat as much at night.

Now you've got the basics. It may seem strange at first to reverse the way you eat your meals, but that's the way you will be able to reverse your life. For anyone with a unique schedule—maybe you work at night and sleep during the day—make your beginning Reverse Diet meal at the beginning of your full day, even if it's at 5 p.m., right before you go to work at 7 p.m. and work through until 4 a.m. Make the Reverse Diet schedule work with your schedule.

3

Reverse Diet Meal Plans and Meal Planning

When I began the Reverse Diet, one of the first things I noticed was how quickly the weight was coming off. That was not only a surprise but a relief, because I've given so much effort on so many other diets with little results. With all the yo-yo dieting I had done, I had never seemed to really lose weight or get healthier. I believe I can do the Reverse Diet for the rest of my life. I can eat normal foods that I actually like and it's easy to prepare them. After four months on the Reverse Diet, I've lost 31 pounds. My beginning weight was 210 pounds and I'm now at 179 pounds. I'm sticking to it. . . . I love it!

—Mark, a successful Reverse Dieter

Reverse Diet Planning and Shopping

As you get into the habit of reversing your meals, you'll find it helpful to reverse some of your other habits, too. In this chapter you will learn a few ways you can make lifestyle adjustments that will help assimilate the plan into your daily life. The Reverse Diet can provide methods to help you plan your meals, prepare your foods, and shop in ways that fit with your schedule and life. Reversing the ways you shop for food and read labels can help you lose weight and change your lifestyle habits for the better. This chapter also includes two full weeks of suggested Reverse Diet meal plans.

One of our clients, Jeanna, said, "Before I planned my meals, I would put off having a large meal in the morning because I felt too rushed to think about it and then I would overeat at lunch and dinner. When I figured out how to plan my breakfast so that it would be quick to prepare, satisfying, and fulfilling, I didn't want to overeat at lunch or at dinner."

Whether you work eight-to-five and have to be up early to get the kids off to school or are at home all day, planning can be something that gives you less of an excuse to give in to bad cravings and choose healthier foods at hand. If you're a spontaneous person and the idea of planning sounds boring to you, reconsider—it will make your life a lot easier because it will free you up to have more time. If you are someone who enjoys planning, you're in luck. When you eat without planning, you're more likely to eat impulsively and to overeat. If you don't plan what to eat and when, you may find yourself influenced not only by your old eating habits but also by your family's food choices or your friends' food choices (if you're joining them for a meal), or you might fall back on fast food and vending machines.

It was clear after interviewing several Reverse Dieters that if they don't plan their meals, they can actually end up eating whatever is in the fridge, ordering in, or going to a convenient restaurant. When you wake up late and haven't planned what you're going to eat, breakfast can become a small snack, lunch a Mexican buffet, and dinner a pepperoni pizza. If you take a little time to plan, this can all be avoided.

Pick a Day to Plan

You don't have to be a planner all day every day—just pick one day a week to do it. For most of our clients, this is Sunday because they work all week or have a full-time job and a family to consider. If you take the time to sit down and plan out your meals for the rest of the week, not only will you eat healthier, you'll also have much more variety rather than just falling back on old standard dishes that you know how to make. They may be easy, but often they are less healthy. Replace them with easier, healthier standards.

When you make a meal plan for the upcoming week, list each day and what you'd like to prepare. Take some time to go through our recipe chapter and choose both some favorites and some recipes that might be new to you. Keeping your menu different will drive away boredom and teach you how to prepare new things. Here is a two-week sample meal plan that Tricia gives her clients when they begin the program. With your own plan, you don't have to put the portion sizes or include this much detail; it can be as simple as "Dinner: Cod Casserole." Portions and extra details are shown here as a guide. Many of the meal plans include dishes with recipes listed in chapter 9, but the recipes yield more than one serving, so use caution.

Two Weeks of Reverse Diet Meal Plans (Weight-Loss Phase)
All Reverse Diet recipes can be found in chapter 9.

WEEK 1

Day 1

Breakfast
> Reverse Diet Egg Bake
> Peach
> 4 ounces of skim milk
> Hot lemon water

Snack
> Celery stalk with fat-free sour cream

Lunch
> 1 cup of whole wheat pasta with olive oil and garlic
> 1 cup of grilled shrimp

Small tossed salad with 2 tablespoons of fat-free dressing

Hot lemon water

Snack

Apple with nonfat yogurt

Dinner

½ cup of shredded wheat and ½ cup of oatmeal with 4 ounces of no-sugar-added cranberry juice

Hot lemon water

Day 2

Breakfast

Baked potato with 1 tablespoon of low-fat, low-sodium butter substitute and 2 tablespoons of fat-free sour cream

½ cup of steamed broccoli with garlic

2 ounces of grilled tofu

Hot lemon water

Snack

¾ ounce of walnuts

Lunch

Reverse Diet Spinach, Strawberry, and Nut Salad

6 ounces of grilled chicken breast

Hot lemon water

Snack

¾ ounce of almonds

Dinner

Reverse Diet Egg Salad Spread

1 slice of whole wheat toast

1 cup of orange juice

Hot lemon water

Day 3

Breakfast

Reverse Diet Chicken Melt

Mashed sweet potato with low-fat, low-sodium butter substitute

Hot lemon water

Snack

Banana

Lunch

Reverse Diet Grumpy Grouper

Steamed asparagus in olive oil and garlic

Hot lemon water

Snack

Rice cake with 1 tablespoon of low-fat, low-sodium peanut butter

Hot lemon water

Dinner

Reverse Diet Tangy Tofu Smoothie

Day 4

Breakfast

Reverse Diet Jambalaya

Hot lemon water

Snack

Reverse Diet Grilled Fruit Kabob

Lunch

Reverse Diet Artichoke Heart Casserole Medley

4 ounces of grilled turkey burger

Hot lemon water

Snack

1½-inch slice of cantaloupe

Dinner

2 eggs, scrambled

Whole wheat toast with low-fat, low-sodium butter substitute

4 ounces of skim milk

Hot lemon water

Day 5

Breakfast

Reverse Diet Eggplant Lasagna

Hot lemon water

Snack

Handful of soy nuts

Lunch

Reverse Diet Chicken Noodle Soup

Sliced tomato

Hot lemon water

Snack

Blueberries and nonfat yogurt

Dinner

Reverse Diet Broccoli, Cauliflower, and Cheese

Reverse Diet Apple Smoothie

Hot lemon water

Day 6

Breakfast

Reverse Diet Veggie Burger, topped with lettuce, tomato, and onion

Slice of whole wheat toast

Hot lemon water

Snack

Reverse Diet Peach and Apple Mash

Lunch

Reverse Diet Stuffed Zucchini

Hot lemon water

Snack

Reverse Diet Raspberry Delight

Dinner

Reverse Diet Chili

Hot lemon water

Day 7

Breakfast

Reverse Diet Southern Fried Chicken

Reverse Diet Potato and Egg Salad

Reverse Diet Coleslaw

Hot lemon water

Snack

¾ cup of mixed fruit salad

Lunch

Reverse Diet Brown Rice and Tuna Casserole

Hot lemon water

Snack

Reverse Diet Cucumber Delights

Dinner

Reverse Diet Banana Split

Hot lemon water

WEEK 2

Day 1

Breakfast

6 ounces of chicken breast

Baked potato with 2 tablespoons of fat-free sour cream

1 cup of broccoli

Hot lemon water

Snack

Peach with nonfat yogurt

Lunch

1 cup of lentil soup

Sliced tomato and onion

Tofu mix ($\frac{1}{2}$ cup of tofu, $\frac{1}{2}$ cup of fat-free sour cream, 1 teaspoon of minced garlic, $\frac{1}{2}$ teaspoon of black pepper, 1 teaspoon of Parmesan cheese)

Hot lemon water

Snack

Handful of unsalted sunflower seeds

Dinner

$\frac{1}{2}$ cup of oatmeal mixed with $\frac{1}{2}$ cup of plain shredded wheat

$\frac{1}{2}$ cup of orange juice poured over cereal mix

Hot lemon water

Day 2

Breakfast

1 cup of whole wheat pasta with Reverse Diet Spaghetti Sauce

Baked tuna steak

French-style green beans with sliced almonds

Hot lemon water

Snack

1 cup of cantaloupe with $\frac{1}{2}$ cup of fat-free cottage cheese

Lunch

Hot lemon water

Roasted red and yellow peppers

Grilled calamari with $\frac{3}{4}$ cup of portabello mushroom

Two slices of grilled tofu

½ cup of orange juice

Snack

Reverse Diet Cucumber Delights

Dinner

2 eggs your way

Slice of whole wheat toast

4 ounces of skim milk

Hot lemon water with mint sprig

Day 3

Breakfast

Hot lemon water

Whole wheat French toast with sugar-free syrup

2 eggs

2 slices of low-sodium turkey bacon

Glass of skim milk

½ cup of orange juice

Snack

½ grapefruit

Lunch

Hot lemon water

Lemon pepper trout

½ cup of corn

Baked sweet potato with 1 tablespoon of low-sodium, low-fat butter substitute

Snack

Reverse Diet Cereal Mix (see dinner, day 1 of week 2)

½ cup of orange juice poured over cereal mix

Dinner

Hot lemon water

2 cups of cooked spinach with ½ tablespoon of olive oil and 1 tablespoon of Parmesan cheese

Day 4

Breakfast

Hot lemon water

4 ounces of broiled London broil

1 cup of whole wheat fettuccine with olive oil and garlic sauce

½ cup of asparagus

Snack

Baked plums with cinnamon

Lunch

Hot lemon water

Baked sliced turkey breast (4 ounces) sandwich on wheat toast

Lettuce

Tomato slice

Sliced onion

Low-fat Swiss cheese

Fat-free Thousand Island dressing

Snack

½ cup of fat-free cottage cheese

1 cup of sliced strawberries

Dinner

Hot lemon water

2 hard-boiled eggs

Reverse Diet Tasty Tofu Dip

Sliced tomatoes

Day 5

Breakfast

Hot lemon water

Veal Parmesan

Baked artichoke hearts with garlic and Reverse Diet Pesto Sauce

1 cup of brown rice lightly buttered and with garlic

Snack

Fat-free yogurt

1 cup of blueberries

Lunch

Hot lemon water

1 cup of shrimp and vegetable soup made with frozen mixed vegetables

Snack

2 celery ribs

2 carrots

2 tablespoons of fat-free blue cheese dressing

¾ cup of low-fat soy milk

Dinner

Hot lemon water

2 ounces of grilled tofu with green beans, watercress, and onions

Day 6

Breakfast

Hot lemon water

4 ounces of grilled chicken breast over 1 cup of baby spinach

½ cup of cherry tomatoes

½ cup of cucumber slices

1 tablespoon of fat-free salad dressing

½ cup of orange juice

Snack

Apple

Lunch

Hot lemon water

Lean ground chuck hamburger

½ whole wheat bun

Grilled green peppers and onions

Sliced tomato

Honey mustard

½ cup of apricots

Snack

Trail mix (½ cup of mini- or bite-size shredded wheat, handful of unsalted peanuts, handful of plain raisins, 2 tablespoons of dried coconut)

Dinner

½ cup of hot lemon water

½ cup of collard greens

½ cup of black-eyed peas

½ cup of chopped onions

2 eggs, scrambled

Day 7

Breakfast

Hot lemon water

4 ounces of calf's liver

½ cup of grilled onions and peppers

Reverse Diet Scalloped Potatoes

Snack

Reverse Diet Cranberry Crush

Lunch

Hot lemon water

Hot banana peppers stuffed with 4 ounces of ground turkey topped with Reverse Diet Spaghetti Sauce

1 ounce of part-skim grated mozzarella and 2 tablespoons of Parmesan cheese

Slice of whole wheat toast with low-fat, low-sodium butter substitute, sprinkled with garlic powder

Snack

½ cup of cherries

½ cup of orange juice

Dinner

Hot lemon water

Sweet potato with low-fat, low-sodium butter substitute and fat-free sour cream

4 ounces of skim milk

Planning briefly one day a week can do wonders for your waistline and any boredom issues you might have with the dishes you typically prepare. If you can't always plan your week in advance, try planning a day's menu the night before, or for dinner during that day's lunch. If you don't usually cook, you may be surprised how much fun you have once you realize that it saves you money and shrinks your clothing size!

Shopping for and Preparing Your Reverse Meals

Here are some tips that will help you plan easily, shop smart, and prep your meals so that they take little time to prepare.

- **Shop smart—and when you have the time.** Try to designate a time to shop when you won't be rushed and can get the right ingredients. If you can, shop when you have time to prepare food afterward. For many this is on Saturday or Sunday morning. If you leave yourself a little time to prepare after you get home from the grocery store, you'll be a lot better off when you want a quick meal during the week.

- **Prepare a list.** Make sure you go to the store with a list. You'll know what you need next and you will be less likely to impulse buy. No need to wander up and down the aisles if you have a list.

- **Don't give in to temptations in the grocery store.** A good way to avoid buying junk food is to go to the store when you're not hungry. Going food shopping at the end of a long workday without having eaten dinner can be tough. You may be tempted to get some old favorite processed foods. Stick to your list and you'll be a lot less likely to grab a bag of Doritos. If you're starving, get an apple from the produce section to eat on the way home. Heidi's been known to grab a bag of green beans and nibble on them in the store, then pay when she gets to the cash register.

- **Avoid two-for-one deals if they aren't really a deal.** A two-for-one sale on a box of frozen beef egg rolls is not really a deal that's going to benefit you. Don't be lured into buying inexpensive processed foods that aren't on the Reverse Diet Food List. As Heidi tells many of her clients, two of a food you didn't need one of is not a bargain—it's a waste of money, calories, and effort.

- **Consciously navigate the grocery store.** You probably have a routine in which you go to the same sections and buy the same foods when you go to the store. You stop at the samples and take one. You go about your shopping half-asleep because you've been to the same store a million times. Wake up! Notice where you're going when you purchase food. Do you get excited when you begin going down the snack food aisle? Avoid it altogether. Do you allow yourself to be suckered in by the foods they put up by the front of the store? They are placed there for a reason; they are the first things you see when you walk in! Ask yourself on your next trip to the grocery store, What can I change about my routine here that will put healthier foods in my kitchen and my body? Becoming a mindful shopper is a helpful step to changing lifestyle habits. If you develop a routine, like fruits and vegetables first, staples second, dairy next, and then frozen, you can beat the other temptations at the store.

- **Get containers for your weekly prep work.** If you don't have any, investing in a good set of Tupperware or the like can be very helpful.

- **Do the prep work early.** When you get home from the grocery store, if you can, wash and cut up all fresh vegetables and put them in containers. That way, you can just take them out and add them to whatever you're cooking. When you want to prepare a meal quickly, your prep time will be minimal. The vegetables will be washed, cut, and dried, and ready to go. If you want to be extra-efficient, go ahead and cook some of the ingredients. If you don't have time to do prep work, buying cut produce is an option. It may seem more expensive, but it's not as expensive as chips and doughnuts in the long term.

- **Buy enough meat for one week at a time.** Unless you have a lot of room in your freezer and want to begin freezing meat, buy only as much as you need. Otherwise, you can freeze it in portion-controlled amounts. Don't get carried away by sales at the butcher shop if you're not freezing extra; otherwise it will go bad. Many of our clients aren't used to shopping for five meals' worth of food, and if a lot of your groceries go bad, you will feel you're wasting money. This can be a deterrent from shopping for groceries and be an incentive for ordering in instead.

- **Prepare your meals the night before.** This is a good thing to do if you don't have time in the morning. Go ahead and cook the whole meal the night before and stick it in the fridge. The next morning, your meal prep will be as easy as grabbing the container and warming it up, and your cleanup time will be a lot less. You'll find it can even be quicker than driving to get fast food.

With this way of preparing meals, not only will you learn how to cook some new dishes, you will begin learning your own tastes better than ever. Along with losing weight, chances are you'll save some money, too. You'll enjoy having more money in the bank when you're ready to go shopping for new clothes!

Avoid Processed Foods

Before Tricia discovered the Reverse Diet, she used to eat processed foods all the time. She and her daughters used to have what they called a "Carby Night." They would pig out on everything they could get their hands on that was processed—canned nacho cheese, boxed dinners, canned meats, fried foods, frozen meals, pizzas, breaded meats, and everything else that they could find that was canned, packaged, frozen, and loaded with sodium or other additives. Nothing was in its natural state. Now that she's been on the Reverse Diet plan for six years, Tricia has lost her taste for processed foods altogether. She'd much rather eat unprocessed, whole food.

Processed foods often contain fructose, dextrose, corn syrup, and other hidden sugars, additives, and preservatives. Hydrogenated oils have lots of sodium. Wrapped in plastic or found in the snack aisle, they are not usually in the produce section. Cheese puffs, nacho chips, and jelly beans are not nutritious and you can eat an entire bag of them and still want more. The further foods get from a recognizable form (whole foods, whole grains, fruits and veggies), the less nutrient-rich they'll be. Where do cream-filled cookies, corn dogs, and snack cakes fit on the food chain? They don't. These are processed foods that won't help you shed your pounds. A whole bag of candy or chips can average upwards of 500 to 1,000 calories! A meal on the Reverse Diet, at breakfast, averages only around 500 to 700 calories.

A more nutrient-rich food choice like a turkey sandwich on whole wheat bread goes a lot further than a candy bar. Instead of spending your calories on refined, processed, starchy carbohydrates, begin choosing whole grain carbohydrates, fruits, vegetables, and lean protein, and you will see that they serve your body better. The table on page 65 shows the nutritional differences between processed foods and more nutritional foods.

As you can see, unprocessed foods usually are more nutritious and satisfying, and they often have fewer calories for more food. A meal of two eggs and toast, even with butter, has fewer calories and more nutrition than one chocolate doughnut.

PROCESSED VERSUS WHOLE FOODS

	Bag of Potato Chips (1-ounce Lays Classic) and a 16-ounce regular soda	Turkey Sandwich (whole wheat bread, 3 ounces meat, tomato, lettuce, 1 teaspoon reduced fat mayonnaise)
Calories	332	279
Total fat	10 grams	4 grams
Saturated fat	3 grams	1 gram
Total carbohydrate	62 grams	27 grams
Protein	2 grams	30 grams
Vitamin A	0%	10%
Vitamin C	10%	14%
Calcium	1%	4%
Iron	3%	17%

	One Chocolate Doughnut	Two Eggs, Slice of Toast, 1 Teaspoon Butter
Calories	250	179
Total fat	12 grams	10 grams
Saturated fat	3 grams	4 grams
Sodium	204 milligrams	211 milligrams
Total carbohydrate	34 grams	14 grams
Protein	3 grams	9 grams

Next time you're in the grocery store or reaching for a snack, think to yourself, Is this a processed food or a whole food? Where does this fit in the food chain? Choose an orange or whole grain bread instead of a pastry, or brown rice, chicken, and veggies over a packaged, frozen TV dinner. Look for foods closest to their natural states. Focus on choosing whole foods that will fill you up, and soon you'll find your taste for processed foods and sugar is almost gone after a few weeks on the Reverse Diet.

REVERSE DIET EXERCISE

Compare Food Lists

Take a moment and grab your journal. Make a list of the processed foods you have a weakness for. Some may be from your trigger food list from chapter 2. How many of these do you consider staples in your diet? Below this list, itemize the foods from the Reverse Diet Food List that you can substitute for these processed foods. Try to stick to those foods until your cravings for processed foods level out.

Reverse Diet Tip

Don't drown your food with processed, high-sodium dressings, sugary ketchup, fatty mayonnaise, or tons of salt. Try learning how to take in the taste and enjoy the food without excessive condiments' overpowering flavor. Use condiments to flavor food slightly rather than to cover up the food's own flavor.

Become Reverse Diet Label Savvy

Researchers have found that one-third of adults surveyed do not generally look at food labels. It's important to become educated in reading labels and know what the unhealthy red flags are. Learning how to read labels is essential to your health and your family's health. Being educated about what ingredients make up the food you eat is one of the most important parts of being healthy for life. Following are some things to look for:

- **Sodium.** Watch the sodium amount and make sure you aren't buying a product that exceeds how much sodium you should have in your daily diet. As noted, you need only 2,300 milligrams of sodium per day. Certain people have to be mindful of their sodium intake more than others—anyone with a history of hypertension or who is over sixty-five. If you stick to the Reverse Diet foods, mainly whole foods and grains, and avoid processed foods, you should be fine. Recognizing the amount of sodium in fast food or processed food can help you see why those foods are particularly unhealthy. (See appendix A.)

One of the main reasons processed foods are so bad is that they contain too much sodium. Did you eat a packaged meat or processed food and retain so much water that even when you stuck to the diet, you didn't lose a pound? Sodium may be the culprit. It's easy to reduce sodium if you avoid processed foods.

Many of our clients who never imagined they would choose a chicken and veggie dish over a fast-food cheeseburger have learned that they like the taste of healthy foods. One client, Marissa, told us after a month on the diet, "I never thought anything could top my favorite burger and fries meal from the local fast-food chain. But I tried the burger and fries after losing 15 pounds on the Reverse Diet plan, and it just tasted salty and gross. I ate half of it and then threw it away." This illustrates that your love of salt and sugar can change, especially if you successfully avoid it for a time.

- **Sugar.** If sugar is one of the first five ingredients on the label, put the item back on the shelf. Avoid high amounts of fructose, dextrose, maltose, high fructose corn syrup, and other corn syrup–hidden sugars ("ose" at the end of an ingredient usually means it's a sugar). The amount on the label should be 5 grams or less per serving. Work on avoiding added sugars. Sugar in and of itself is not bad, but if it's the main ingredient on a label, that is a red flag that indicates the food most likely will have a lot of calories and probably not a lot of nutrition. Sugar has 16 calories per teaspoon—get used to using less and reversing your taste for sweetness. Nonnutritive sweeteners may be lower in calories, but they can also keep your sweet tooth going.

- **Additives and preservatives.** These are no-no's! Avoid them as much as possible. The Reverse Diet is about focusing on eating unprocessed whole foods.

- **Anything with more than three or four wholesome ingredients.**

These are off limits. Most likely they have multiple ingredients that aren't nutritious because they've been highly processed.

- **Trans fat.** Avoid this when possible. Trans fat is found wherever you see the phrase "partially hydrogenated vegetable oil," primarily in vegetable shortenings, many margarines, processed foods, doughnuts, commercially prepared foods (especially fast-food french fries), cookies, cakes, fried foods, and many commercial snack foods. Trans fat does not inhibit weight loss per se, but it does contribute to increased LDL ("bad") cholesterol levels. When LDL levels are high, you are at greater risk of heart disease.

- **Saturated fat and cholesterol.** All the labels that are FDA regulated have a Daily Value percentage, abbreviated as % DV. For both saturated fat and cholesterol, look for 5 percent or less; 20 percent or more is too high.

REVERSE DIET EXERCISE

Check Out Food Labels Carefully

For the next two weeks, check every label of every food you purchase or regularly eat. Read labels so that eventually it will be a habit to look and know immediately how much fat, sodium, and sugar you can expect from certain foods.

Remember, reading labels is important—but also remember that the more unlabeled and unpackaged, produce-type food you buy, the better. You don't have to check for trans fat or sodium on a head of broccoli or lettuce.

Nutrition Facts	
Serving Size 1 cup (228g)	
Servings Per Container 2	

Amount Per Serving	
Calories 260	Calories from Fat 120

	% Daily Value*
Total Fat 13g	**20%**
Saturated Fat 5g	**25%**
Trans Fat 0g	
Cholesterol 30mg	**10%**
Sodium 660mg	**28%**
Total Carbohydrate 31g	**10%**
Dietary Fiber 0g	**0%**
Sugars 5g	
Protein 5g	

Vitamin A 4%	•	Vitamin C 2%
Calcium 15%	•	Iron 4%

* Percent Daily Values are based on a 2,000 calorie diet. Your Daily Values may be higher or lower depending on your calorie needs:

		Calories:	2,000	2,500
Total Fat	Less than		65g	80g
Sat Fat	Less than		20g	25g
Cholesterol	Less than		300mg	300mg
Sodium	Less than		2,400mg	2,400mg
Total Carbohydrate			300g	375g
Dietary Fiber			25g	30g

Calories per gram:
Fat 9 • Carbohydrate 4 • Protein 4

The Carbohydrate Myth

Carbohydrates are not all created equal. Under the influence of the recent low-carb fad, many subscribe to the myth that all carbohydrates are bad. They are not. Carbohydrates have been demonized in our weight-conscious media, but it's best if you begin to think this way: It's not foods you eat that are bad—it's your eating habits.

That said, you don't have to have a degree in nutrition to know that certain foods are better for you than others.

The confusion in the past few years over which is better, protein or carbohydrate, is misguided. Both are imperative for optimal performance and health; they do different things in your body. Carbohydrate fuels your muscle and may bolster immune function after heavy exertion, and whole grain, fruit, and vegetable carbohydrates carry vitamins, minerals, and phytochemicals along for the ride. Protein's role is tissue repair, hormone synthesis, and enzyme formation as well as immune function.

The term *carbohydrate* actually covers a broad category that includes vegetables; fruits; beans; whole grains such as whole wheat bread, brown rice, and whole wheat pasta; and other nutrient-rich foods as well as sugar-laden candy, cookies, ice cream, chips and other carbs. Reverse Dieters are encouraged, as you see on the Reverse Diet Food List, to eat whole grains and lots of vegetables and fruit, and avoid refined carbohydrates. The rule is, the more refined and processed, the less fulfilling and nutrient-rich. Usually the starchy, sugary carbs are the ones you learn to crave. You may eat a large amount of them but you'll never feel full and satisfied—instead you just want to eat more. Processed carbs like cheese puffs, snack cakes and other sweets are calorie-rich but nutrient-poor.

There are many advantages to eating complex, less-processed starches and grains:

- They contain more vitamins and minerals.
- They are higher in fiber.
- They are a great energy source.

- They provide a more even energy release.
- They provide a moderate protein contribution.

If you find that your weight fluctuates a lot with carbohydrates, it may be because you store 2 grams of water for every gram of carbohydrate you eat and store. If you've ever avoided carbs, lost a few pounds, and then eaten, say, a potato and felt like you've gained 2 pounds, it was water weight (unless you had nacho cheese, bacon, and sour cream on top!).

Foods such as carrots, potatoes, and corn are really considered starches although technically they are vegetables. A sweet potato is probably one of the most nutrient-rich foods but is more caloric than, say, spinach. So when you are planning a day, don't fall into thinking you ate your vegetables because you had french-fried sweet potatoes. Go for the greens daily, orange at least every other day. And count carrots, peas, corn, and potatoes among grains and starches instead of vegetables.

Tips on Pasta Prep

There are ways to prepare carbs such as pasta so that you can enjoy the food without it dominating your entire meal. Many clients think two cups of pasta is a normal serving. It isn't. In actuality, 1 cup is a more appropriate portion for most people. One good way to make a better, well-rounded meal is to make the pasta serving smaller, 1 cup, and add other nutrient-rich whole foods, such as protein and vegetables, to it.

Pasta with chicken and broccoli in a red sauce or shrimp and arugula in a broth are both good examples of healthy, nutritious food combinations. The issue is not the pasta or carbs; the issue is the amount and way in which they are eaten. Try whole wheat pasta, which will provide fiber and make you feel satisfied even in smaller portions. Pay attention to the ingredients that make up your meals and try to have an even variety, not all carbs. Prepare equal parts pasta, vegetables, and protein, and a salad. When you mix whole wheat pasta with proteins and vegetables, you'll feel more satisfied after you've eaten your meal because your body's nutritional needs are being met.

Reverse Diet Tip

A study recently found that broth and soup actually make people feel fuller than beverages do. Try making soup when you want to be satisfied with less.

Hydrating—the Reverse Way

The Reverse Diet has a unique take on hydrating. The amount of water you drink has to do with what you need specifically for your body and lifestyle. You don't necessarily have to drink eight to ten glasses of water. The amount of water you need depends on your own personal bodily needs. A small person needs less than someone who is 6'4" and weighs over 200 pounds, for example. Becoming properly hydrated isn't necessarily limited to water; it can also include drinking tea, milk, juice, soup, Sunshine Tea, and other liquids (except alcohol and coffee) that contribute to your hydration in a healthy way. If you are an avid exerciser, obviously you will need more than someone who does not exercise. If you live in a hot climate and you find yourself outdoors often, you will need more than someone who sits at a desk all day. Figuring out how much water you need each day is a personal decision. We don't want you forcing liquids, but it is true that many people walk around moderately dehydrated, which can be accompanied by headaches, nausea, and fatigue. Since water is a part of every single cell membrane and metabolic process in the body, paying attention to hydration is worth it.

When you feel thirsty, you're already dehydrated. Some interpret thirst as hunger. Being thirsty is a message from your body that you haven't had enough fluids. If you find you're thirsty often, that should be a clue to drink more water and other healthy liquids regularly. If you're never thirsty and you feel you take in a decent amount of healthy fluids, you're probably fine with the amount of water you drink. As we age, however, our thirst mechanism is less precise, so drink water regularly to make sure you are in the habit of hydrating your body. If your urine is dark or looks like apple juice, you are probably dehydrated. If it is in good volume and pale yellow, you are probably hydrated.

The Benefits of Sunshine Tea

Reverse Dieters drink what we call Sunshine Tea, which is simply hot lemon water. Tricia began drinking it, and it has become one of her Reverse Diet staples. She used to drink soda all the time; now she drinks Sunshine Tea and she recommends it to all her clients. It's incredibly easy to make. It's your choice to use fresh lemons or bottled lemon juice.

Fresh: Just boil or heat water, slice a fresh lemon, and squeeze a few slices into your cup.

Bottled: Presqueezed lemon juice is fine, just make sure it is low in sodium. Use two to four tablespoons to a cup, to taste.

These are the benefits of Sunshine Tea that we've found so far:

- It promotes bowel movements and controls constipation and diarrhea by eliminating waste more efficiently.
- It's a good source of vitamin C.
- Water enhances the beauty of your skin. Drinking the lemon juice rejuvenates the skin from within thanks to vitamin C.
- It replaces your need for hot beverages such as tea or coffee.
- It is soothing to sip. It can help slow you down and take the edge off your hunger.

We encourage you to use Sunshine Tea instead of caffeine in the mornings. Even if it seems strange at first to snuggle up with a piping hot mug of Sunshine Tea instead of your standard coffee, tea, Frappucino, or hot chocolate, it will become a taste you enjoy.

You'll notice it is relaxing to sip instead of gulp a beverage. When one sips a tea or water, it forces one to slow down. In the time it takes to consume a cup of warm tea, the edge can be taken off anxiety or a compulsion to eat—and that will help you with weight-loss efforts.

Cut Back on Caffeine

Most of our clients don't want to hear it if they're in the caffeine camp, but it's worth considering the pros and cons of caffeine. Maybe it's become something you don't think you can live without. Part of the Reverse Diet is rethinking habit-forming consumption. Are you addicted to caffeine? If so, do you drink too much of it— more than one or two cups a day? Some people use caffeine like a drug, as a substitute for snacks, or to help them through long stretches without food.

One client, Josie, would have a cup of coffee or soda when she was hungry instead of a snack. Essentially she was using it to mask her hunger. Reverse Dieters should listen when they're hungry and feed their body appropriate amounts of healthy food, so masking hunger with caffeine is not something the plan endorses. Disguising the messages your body is sending you is not healthy. When you are not listening to your body, you are at a greater risk of overeating. Whether by starving yourself or overeating, you are sabotaging your ultimate goal.

If you do decide to drink caffeine, do it sparingly. Here are a few things you should know about caffeine:

- It doesn't boost long-term energy. You may get a temporary pick-me-up but you may also crash at the end of the day. If you find yourself using caffeine as a crutch in the afternoon, recognize you may need more sleep at night. Also, drinking caffeine at night or within five hours of sleep can compound sleeping problems.

- It doesn't help you lose weight. Studies indicate that large amounts of caffeine consumption a day (six or more cups) may help with weight loss initially, but that loss is not significant or permanent. There's also no evidence that increasing caffeine intake alone has any effect on weight loss; you have to eat a healthy diet and preferably exercise for permanent weight loss.

- Although caffeine has been shown to interfere with calcium absorption, this can be counterbalanced by adding even a splash of milk to your cup of java.

If you do decide to give up the caffeine, it may be a bit painful at first, but after the withdrawal is over you'll feel the relief of waking up in the morning and being free of the craving for it. Looking for longer-lasting energy sources is a good idea regardless of whether you continue to drink caffeine in moderation or not. We're not just talking short-term goals; the Reverse Diet is about long-term lifestyle changes.

Tricia has experienced dramatic energy increases since she replaced her favorite soda with Sunshine Tea. Anyone who knows her personally will tell you that she is full of energy all day long. She's helped her clients be the same. Though they might get headaches for a few days after giving up caffeine, once that passes they are all so glad they gave it up! If you're not big on lemon or lemon flavoring, try green tea in place of a caffeinated beverage in the morning and see how it feels. Green tea has ⅓ less caffeine than coffee, and it contains beneficial antioxidants.

Enjoy Savory Nuts

Nuts provide antioxidants and phytonutrients that are heart healthy. They provide protein, fiber, iron, calcium, vitamin E, arginine, magnesium, copper, potassium, and folic acid along with tocopherols and plant sterols, all of which are heart healthy. The fat in nuts is unsaturated—a healthier type of fat. Just 1 ounce (a handful) four or five times a week is recommended to help maintain a healthy blood pressure and arterial function. Regular intake of nuts is recommended as part of the DASH diet (Dietary Advances to Stop Hypertension). In moderation, nuts are absolutely part of a heart-healthy diet. On the Reverse Diet, we encourage you to be a nut about nuts.

Consume Calcium-Rich Foods

You have probably heard by now about the importance of calcium for bone health and how many of us still fail to reach the recommended intake each day. Considering that osteoporosis affects over 10 million Americans, we recommend that everyone take a multivitamin/mineral supplement (men, and women who do not menstruate, should take one without iron) and a calcium supplement.

We all know the benefits of consuming adequate calcium—strong bones and a decreased risk of osteoporosis and stress fractures. But calcium also can help to reduce symptoms of premenstrual syndrome, help maintain a healthy blood pressure, and decrease your risk of colon cancer.

Then why aren't we getting enough? Most Americans don't get the recommended amount of calcium-rich foods to meet their needs. Aim for 1,000 to 1,200 milligrams a day. It has become much easier for us to up our intake of calcium. We don't have to rely on only dairy to meet our needs. Besides the many supplements or antacids that provide calcium, many food manufacturers have been adding calcium to their foods as well.

Talk to your health professional about taking a calcium supplement. Weight loss can take a toll on bone health; there is a loss of bone while on calorie-restricted plans. Be sure to counterbalance this loss by including dairy daily in your diet even while losing weight. Remember that along with calcium, other nutrients such as vitamin D and magnesium are crucial for bone health. Check out appendix B for more information on calcium supplements and how much calcium is in your yogurt and tofu and other food sources.

The Ring Test

One great example of pinpointing what's happening in your body and seeing the effects of processed food is Tricia's ring test. Tricia noticed when she ate processed foods with a high salt content, she retained water. Journaling was a major key to discovering this. She would weigh herself and eventually could see that salt affected her the very next day. She developed what she calls the ring test: "If I wake up in the morning and my rings are tight, salt is the culprit. After watching my body on the Reverse Diet plan for so long, I found the ring test was a necessity!"

Sodium can make you feel bloated. Using too much salt can also hide subtle flavors in whole foods. As you continue to read the signals your body sends, you will become more and more adept at figuring out how processed foods, additives, and sodium affect you.

An Alternative to Processed Sweets

Many Reverse Dieters have found they can kick their sweet cravings with one of Tricia's Reverse Diet recipes, which can serve as a dessert.

Tricia's Special Cereal

½ cup mini- or bite-size shredded wheat

½ cup uncooked oatmeal

4 ounces orange juice or no-sugar-added cranberry juice

Mix together and enjoy.

One Reverse Dieter, Mandy, reported, "I can honestly say that the oatmeal, shredded wheat, and OJ mix cuts down cravings for sugar for me." Whole grain cereal boosts your energy, is high in fiber and nutrients, and gives you a full feeling longer than processed, sugary carbs do.

Heidi often encourages her clients to have fruit instead of processed sweets. An apple or an orange will begin to taste better than most candy if you start working them into your daily diet. Natural sugars can be the most satisfying, without the sugar highs and lows of processed sugar.

Don't Fall for the All-or-Nothing Approach

Our food consciousness is groomed by many of the popular diets that exclude bread, pasta or potatoes, or sugar or have specific combinations of foods. This cult of modern diets fosters an unhealthy attitude that sets us up for disaster: the all-or-nothing mind-set.

When you say, "I'm never eating cookies again," most likely you can't stop thinking about eating cookies and eventually will eat one (and probably many more) again. When you make an agreement with yourself that you probably will not keep, you are setting yourself up for failure. One of the reasons the anti-carb diets don't work is that eventually you will be eating carbs again. Adopting the all-or-nothing mind-set is not a way to change your lifestyle. Focusing on what you can have instead of what you can't have is a better way to navigate life changes. Being mindful of what you eat rather than being absolute about what you cannot eat will get you much further.

Reverse Diet Tips

- Planning will save you time in the long run—you'll be more able to stick to the Reverse Diet plan without veering off track with unplanned meals and snacks along the way.
- Pick a day to plan and leave time to shop and prep your meals.
- When you're in the grocery store, read labels carefully. Make sure you check out the labels on foods you usually pick up that you never closely examined before.
- Remember, large amounts of sodium come from processed foods—even more than the average person adds to his or her food.

Reverse Diet Portions— and Plateaus

At seventy years old, it's not so easy to lose weight. I went to the doctor to get a checkup and he told me that I had high cholesterol and I needed to lose some weight. I heard about the Reverse Diet Web site. Tricia was great, and she helped me with everything. I now cook all of my meals myself. After six months, my cholesterol and blood pressure were reduced. My doctor said I looked a lot better. And I lost 40 pounds! I breathe easier, too. The Reverse Diet has added years to my life!

—Fanny, a successful Reverse Dieter

Make Changes in Your Life to Make Changes in Your Body

As you follow the Reverse Diet one day at a time, one week at a time, it's a good idea to focus not only on changing your meals, but on how you think your choices affect your body.

Reverse Portion Distortion

It's important to pay attention to the size of your portions. Many Reverse Dieters come to us with the impression that a diet is a form of deprivation. They may starve, binge, skip meals, and try to eat as little as possible to lose weight. For these dieters, losing weight *is* deprivation. But it doesn't have to be.

On the Reverse Diet, while you are never deprived of food—you get to eat like a queen or king first thing in the morning—subtle shifts in perception take place, especially with your expectations of portions. When clients are initially introduced to the Reverse Diet, they are encouraged to rethink what they consider deprivation and portion size. Are we really meant to eat gigantic portions at every meal? The Reverse Diet says no. Large portions have become a way of life rather than something necessary to our health and well-being.

In our society, big portions are associated with good value. Many restaurants serve extra-large portions because it's what their customers expect. We are a supersized nation. A study published in the *Journal of the American Dietetic Association* indicates that portion sizes of restaurants and packaged foods have increased substantially during the past twenty years, especially when compared to the initial introduction of these products.

There are so many reasons that larger portions have become part of the American way of life. One of them is that as a culture, we can financially afford large portions. All of this leads to what experts call *portion distortion*. Bear in mind that portions in packaged foods have increased over the years. For example, a Hershey bar started out as 6 ounces and is now as big as 8 ounces; a soda at McDonald's started out as 7 ounces and is now as large as 64 ounces!

At home, families encourage kids to clean their plates. Part of this comes from a natural urge to nurture. A huge amount of food is seen as an extension of love. But allowing kids to eat whatever they want when they want and providing abundant food because parents feel unlimited love for their children promotes obesity. If you love your children, isn't it a good idea to teach them to have a healthier relationship with food?

A jumbo muffin is equal to ten slices of bread, a standard pasta dish has two or more cups. It's very important to become aware of how much starch you eat at one time. The average person should limit starch consumption to 2 to 3 cups per day. That may seem like a small amount—but in reality it's an appropriate amount. It is the amount of starch your body needs in a day (more about this later in this chapter), unless you are a very active athlete, regardless of what you emotionally or habitually have come to want. On the Reverse Diet, we encourage 1½ or more cups of starch in the form of whole grains a day. This can take the form of ½ cup of pasta or rice, one slice of bread, or ¾ cup of cereal. Each of these portions constitutes one serving, and we recommend you have three whole grains a day.

With the Reverse Diet, we reverse our portion expectations. If you perceive that you are being deprived at certain times during the day such as dinner, you will have difficulty staying on the diet or being satisfied emotionally, even if your body is satisfied. If you come to understand portions appropriate for what your body needs, you will begin to eat only what you can burn off. When you tune in to hunger, satiety, and grades of fullness, when you give yourself permission to eat healthfully and to stop when you are full with the knowledge that you can eat again when you are hungry again, you will lose weight. Learning to listen to your body signals will help you know how big your portions should be. Some days you may want two slices of bread and on other days one will do.

REVERSE DIET EXERCISE

Stop Portion Distortion

Take a moment with your journal. Imagine you are getting ready to eat a meal in a restaurant or in your home and you get to choose the portion size. Try to re-create what your typical automatic thoughts are. Which of these ways do you think?

I want as much as I can fit on my plate because I'm starving! I'm going to eat everything I can get my hands on—and I don't care what it is.

Or:

I'm going to start out with a little, eat it slowly, and enjoy every bite, and then eventually I might eat more if I'm still hungry.

What is your internal dialogue when you are deciding how much you're going to eat? Listen to your automatic thoughts when you sit down to your next meal.

Reverse Dieters work on changing their portion distortion especially at dinnertime so they won't feel deprived when they give themselves only what is a healthy portion. By reducing the typical amount of food you put on your plate at first and then eating slowly to enjoy the food, followed by getting seconds *only* if you are still really hungry, you will usually eat less and feel better about yourself. If you are still hungry, eat seconds as long as it's a legitimate response to hunger. You won't have that awful guilty feeling. Imagine—you can feel full, satisfied, and proud of yourself at the end of a meal. On the Reverse Diet, calorie counting is not mandatory; rather, we would like you to be mindful of portion size and balanced meals.

Portions Are Personal

Like everything else on the Reverse Diet, much of it is about what works for you. Eliminate high-calorie, low-nutrient foods like sodas, pastries, sweets, and cakes. Eat moderate amounts of starchy carbohydrates like potatoes and brown rice.

Choose portions suited for your body type and your weight goal. Notice your body type and the amount of food you are eating. If you are 6'3", you're going to eat a larger portion than if you were 5'5". Similarly, notice your portions in relation to how much you wish to lose.

At the same time, remember to distribute calories throughout the day. For example, instead of having all your high-calorie, higher-carb foods at once, have them throughout the day. Two cups a day can be distributed into ½ cup at breakfast, ½ cup at lunch, ½ cup as part of a snack, and ½ cup at dinner.

Have some carbs at breakfast time. It may seem strange at first, but many of our clients enjoy whole wheat pasta, brown rice, a baked potato, oatmeal, a whole grain waffle, or whole grain cereal in the morning, and it's a perfect way to fuel yourself through a busy day.

As one Reverse Dieter, Rick, said, "I never thought I'd want chicken, veggies, and rice, or pasta and shrimp first thing in the morning, I was not even used to eating breakfast, and sometimes I'd skip lunch. Now that I have the hang of eating a big breakfast, I have all sorts of dinner things in the morning and don't miss them in the evening. I *really* don't miss the awful pig-out dinner sessions I'd have after not eating breakfast or lunch." If you think about it, this style of eating gives you *more* choices.

Understand that there is a difference between "serving sizes," the standard sizes for measuring used on food labels, and what you actually eat or what is served to you in a restaurant. For instance, a restaurant might give you three "servings" of pasta, but what you eat is your "portion." In the Reverse Diet, we don't assign specific portions to you. We firmly believe you should choose your portions as they relate to your hunger levels and your own personal Hunger Scale. Your portion should be based on how hungry you truly are. We recommend, though, that you pay attention to the balance in your meal so that the meal is not all starch or all protein. It helps to be familiar with what standard serving sizes are as a starting point to rounding out meals.

It also helps to have an image of what standard serving sizes look like. That way, in your mind's eye, if a label says six servings, you'll know how much food that is. Size up the serving size with an easy-to-remember visual. These are some of the examples used by the USDA:

Portion	*Looks Like*
½ cup fruit, vegetable, cooked cereal, pasta, or rice	a small fist
3 ounces of cooked meat, poultry, or fish	a deck of cards
1 tortilla	a small (7-inch) plate
½ bagel	the diameter of a large coffee lid

1 muffin	a large egg
1 teaspoon of margarine or butter	a thumb tip
2 tablespoons of peanut butter	a golf ball
a small baked potato	a computer mouse
1 pancake or waffle	a four-inch CD
1 medium apple or orange	a baseball
4 small cookies (e.g., vanilla wafers)	four casino chips
1½ ounces of cheese	6 dice

When to Weigh Yourself

While we don't think weighing is the be-all and end-all to finding out if you're a success or not, we do encourage getting on the scale once or twice a week in the first phase so that you can get a handle on what works for you and what doesn't. If you're successful on the Reverse Diet right away, knowing that you have just lost some weight is a great incentive to stay on the program. And once you have lost weight, monitoring when you have gained two pounds and getting back on track is essential for long-term success.

Weigh three times a week only if you are impatient. We advise against it, though. Do not weigh every day; it can sabotage your motivation. People who weigh too often are unrealistic in their weight-loss expectations. They can set themselves up for disaster when they find their bodies don't react in a predictable manner day to day.

If you stick to a normal workweek schedule, it might be best to avoid weighing on the weekends and weigh only during the week. Monday and Thursday are the days that Tricia does it. If Tuesday or Friday works better for you, that's fine. On Monday (or Tuesday) you can record your weight. Those who have shift schedules should weigh on their version of Monday. Whatever the day, it's a good idea to weigh first thing in the morning after you wake and urinate.

The workweek is best because often we are not on our typical eating schedule on the weekend. You may have one weekday routine and another weekend routine, both of which give you Reverse Diet structure. Weekends are when more high-risk times might present themselves, and it may be more difficult to adhere to your new, healthier regime. With the kids at home and events like parties, picnics, reunions, and gatherings, it can be hard to regulate all the time.

Whatever you do, do not live by the scale. Make sure that weighing is not the only way you judge your success. Many other things go into your overall body image and healthy lifestyle beyond weight. Pay attention to how your clothes feel, how your energy level is climbing, and how much healthier you feel in general.

Body Composition

Heidi encourages her clients to use the scale as one piece of information but also to recognize that body weight is not the same as body composition. Your body is made up of fat, muscle, and bone. Two people who weigh 140 pounds may have very different bodies. One might have more muscle (which weighs more than fat) and be more fit overall, and the other might have more fat. Muscle is important not only because it burns more calories but also because it supports your posture and general health. As people lose weight, they often lose fat and muscle. When they regain the weight, they gain back fat but not muscle, unless they are exercising and weight lifting.

Your muscle is also called *lean mass*. You want your lean mass to be as high as it can be. As we age, we lose lean mass naturally. It is important to incorporate exercise into our routines because if we exercise and lift weights as we age, we can maintain our lean active muscle tissue and eat a healthy amount while maintaining a healthy weight. Each time you lose weight, you are in danger of losing muscle; the trick is to lose weight by healthy means so that you can retain as much muscle as possible. That means eating appropriate amounts and whole foods at the right times of day while you stay active.

The Plateau

Inevitably, after you've been losing weight for a while, your scale will stop moving in the direction you want it to before you reach your goal. This is completely normal. Almost every Reverse Dieter has experienced it. Plateaus happen for several reasons. One reason is that as your body becomes smaller, it adapts to and needs fewer calories—a larger body uses more calories than a smaller body does. It now needs to readjust the thermostat for the new, lower weight. Your body's engine is idling sometimes rather than actively dropping pounds. When this happens, if you maintain your action steps and a healthy eating plan, your body will resume its healthy eating habits and you'll start to lose more weight.

In the first week of a plateau, look at your journal for the past five days and answer these questions:

- Have you eaten the foods on the Reverse Diet Food List as consistently as you could?
- Have you eaten your meals as you should, in big, medium, and small portions?
- Have your mealtimes been approximately consistent?
  - For breakfast, this means eating within an hour of waking.
  - For dinner it means eating three hours or more before bedtime, but be careful: if you eat more than four hours before, you may be hungry before going to bed. In that case, try just a piece of fruit to bridge the hunger gap until morning.
- Have you overeaten during the week? If so, try the Reverse Buster Diet for two days (page 142).
- Have you skipped any meals?

If you have followed the Reverse Diet and feel secure, wait a week while continuing to follow the plan. Sometimes the plateau will continue for a limited amount of time and eventually it will break on its own. Here are some other options to consider:

- Carefully look at what you've been consuming. Have you been eating as much food as you ate at your old weight even though you might be 30 pounds lighter now? If so, you may need to reduce your portions just a little to reflect what your now smaller body needs.

- Another option is to step up your physical activity or exercise. Read more about this in chapter 7.

- You can post your five-day menu on the Reverse Diet Web site and others will help you to see if you need to add or reduce foods or delete others.

Retune In to Your Body

Mindful attention to your body, emotions, and environment is a consistent theme on the Reverse Diet. If you learn how to retune in to your body, you'll recognize whether you're really hungry or not. You'll also notice your new body's needs as opposed to the amount of food or calories you consumed at your old weight.

Understanding what your body needs and overcoming your own internal dialogue of habitual eating will help you see why you continue to lose weight and what's actually happening when you don't. You may also notice how processed foods make you feel and how well your body responds when you stick to whole, nutritious foods. When you're tuned in to your body and are truly aware of its signals, you will find that your body does best when you feed it the Reverse Diet foods at the right times of day. As so many successful Reverse Dieters will tell you, your body will thank you by becoming a body you can be proud of.

REVERSE DIET EXERCISE

Deal with Portions and Plateaus

- Examine your portion distortion over the next few days. When you automatically want a certain amount of food, is it because you are truly hungry or because you're just used to eating that much at a time? Recognize, however, that some days you may be hungrier than other days.

- Make sure you're recording your meals and reactions to those meals in your journal.

- If you plateau, carefully look over your journal and see what the real reason might be.

Reverse Diet Success

When I began the Reverse Diet, I had heart palpitations and fluttering and I was under a lot of stress. I went to a cardiologist. The doctor told me that for a woman of my height, 5'2", I was way too heavy at 240 pounds and that my health was compromised. For breakfast I had caffeine (a large coffee from Dunkin' Donuts) with an onion bagel with cream cheese. I had a McDonald's burger and fries for lunch (supersized with a large Diet Coke). The doctor's visit was my wake-up call.

I saw Tricia and Heidi on *Good Morning America*. From there I searched the Internet and found a news article by Wendy Bell from the Pittsburgh channel. It had Tricia's shopping list and menus. I started the next day, May 20th. Almost two weeks later I had lost 19 pounds. From there I started to lose 2 pounds a week and then 1 to 2 pounds a week. I am down 50 pounds now, and I weigh 190 pounds.

The plan is very easy to follow and the recipes are delicious. So fill up your freezer with fruits, vegetables, fish, and chicken—and start your day off with a delicious big breakfast!

—Meagan, a successful Reverse Dieter

5

Reverse Diet Motivation: Dealing with High-Risk Moments

When I began the Reverse Diet at 189 pounds, I immediately began losing weight. After losing the first 30 pounds, I had the energy to be more active. Now that I've lost 50 pounds, I can be even more active. I played basketball with my husband and two children yesterday for an hour, and it was exhilarating. I feel better emotionally, too, when I don't feed my moods with food. Now I can do things with my family I couldn't do before and I don't have the ever-present guilt that accompanies low energy and overeating. I've got the whole family on the Reverse Diet now. Thank you!

—Lindsey, a successful Reverse Dieter

As you get into the habit of reversing your meals and focusing on eating mostly whole foods, you'll begin to work toward overcoming other challenges that stand in the way of success, whether they are motivational, emotional, or environmental. While you are on the Reverse Diet, your weight changes will be longer lasting if you learn to overcome the things that set off poor eating cycles. When you begin pinpointing your obstacles, you can better anticipate them and plan a way around or through them. Take a close look at your food journal—when are your high-risk times? Being mindful of triggers that motivate you to overeat will help you succeed on the Reverse Diet.

Preventing Overeating: When Are Your High-Risk Moments?

We hope you've been keeping a journal with great detail since beginning the program. It bears repeating: if you are honest in your journal, you will be able to see where, when, and how to prevent overeating tendencies. Very often those overeating episodes have a pattern; they occur at high-risk times throughout the day. Pinpointing high-risk moments is essential to learning about and changing your eating habits for the better.

REVERSE DIET EXERCISE

When Are You Vulnerable?

Take a look at your journal. When are the times you've overeaten since you've been on the Reverse Diet? We all have our particular moment in which we are most vulnerable. If you know when you usually overeat, you can start taking steps to anticipate and prevent or change that pattern. If you haven't been as descriptive as possible about the times when you have slipped up because you're just getting the hang of it, think about the last time you ate too big a portion, or when you ate foods that are not on the Reverse Diet Food List. What time of day was it? What were the circumstances surrounding that particular instance?

Falling Off the Reverse Diet Wagon

When are your high risk-times? Maybe you realize that when everyone in the office orders from your favorite Mexican restaurant, you can't resist the deep-fried chicken chimichangas. It's the middle of the day at work, when you have a million things coming at you at one time—the phone won't stop ringing, you have a deadline to meet, you think you'll be at the office until seven that evening—and finally, a coworker pops his head in the door and asks if you'd like your usual from La Hacienda. With a one-track mind you think to yourself, a moment to relax, a moment to indulge, a moment to eat unabashedly as you'd like and leave the rest behind. Only this once . . .

In a nutshell, that is a high-risk moment.

Here are some examples of high-risk times for some Reverse Dieters. You might overeat when you are:

- Bored
- Lonely
- Sad
- Stressed-out
- Angry
- Anxious
- Tired
- Misunderstood
- Frustrated
- Emotionally drained
- Out of control
- Feeling isolated
- Feeling overwhelmed
- Experiencing low self-esteem
- Going out to eat after a long, hard day at work
- On the way to a big meeting for work and are on edge
- Having a fight with a family member
- At a buffet
- Passing a bakery or a chocolate shop
- Going to your in-laws' house and feeling nervous, anxious, or angry
- Going out with a friend who always eats unhealthy food and encourages you to do the same

- Going to dinner after drinking alcohol
- Just home from work and too tired to cook so you order fast food in
- Going to a party or a special occasion
- Experiencing something stressful with your job—good or bad (e.g., promotion or demotion)
- Having dinner with your family when they do not want to be on the Reverse Diet plan
- Being pressured by your family or friends to eat unhealthy foods
- At an event or an outing (e.g., sporting event or concert)
- On vacation

When you pig out or choose foods that aren't healthy, it's not the most terrible thing in the world, because even though it is something you are trying to prevent, it gives you an opportunity to examine why you are overeating.

It is normal to occasionally fall off the wagon and slip up in your meal plan. Admitting it helps you deal with the consequences and see clearly why you did what you did. Instead of feeling guilt and remorse, use the experience to figure out how to alter the course next time. Don't focus on your bad feelings after overeating and avoid blanket statements, such as "I'll never eat cookies again." Instead, focus on "I won't let myself get so hungry that I can't make a healthy decision about what to eat. Next time, I will eat a healthy snack when I notice that I am hungry." The Reverse Diet encourages you to figure out how to read the signals and be prepared for them.

As one of our clients, Brenda, said, "I am wearing pants that I have not been able to wear for three years. I follow the principle of the program, but one important thing I have learned is that if I eat something off my plan, I don't beat myself up about it. I say, okay, it happens, now I need to get back on the program."

This is exactly the attitude to have. If you feel terrible and beat yourself up, you are more prone to fall into negative thought patterns—the very same patterns that contributed to overeating and weight gain in the first place. You want to avoid or change those patterns to get the weight off. The key is to get over the incident and begin figuring out why it happened so you can prevent it happening again. Studies have shown that people who maintain healthy weight balances are able to be consistent in their eating patterns even on weekends, holidays, and special events, and also get back on track quickly after regaining a pound or two if they overeat. Don't dwell on the fact that you ate the wrong thing or use it as a license to eat more—get back on the Reverse Diet.

For those who don't want to slow down on their weight-loss process and who want to avoid setbacks due to overeating episodes, Tricia has developed a remedy, the Reverse Buster. It is more restrictive than the basic Reverse Diet Food List, but if you want to really reverse a recent episode of falling off the wagon, try it. More about the Reverse Buster can be found in chapter 6.

What to Do Instead of Overeating

Troubleshooting your danger zones involves making subtle changes in your habits so that you give yourself room for another, healthier alternative food choice. Try to change your internal dialogue, and see the situation for what it is. Think about the repercussions.

When you face cravings, however they are triggered, troubleshoot with options other than overeating. It's really like impulse control. Cravings often last about 20 to 30 minutes, so if you can divert your attention for that time you may find that the craving subsides. Some of the things the Reverse Diet recommends include:

- Drinking a lot of water
- Eating a bowl of Tricia's Reverse Diet Cereal (see page 186)
- Walking with a friend, with the dog, or alone
- Window shopping—but not in a grocery store
- Journaling
- Calling or writing to a friend
- Washing your face
- Brushing your teeth

- Doing yoga
- Meditation
- Listening to music
- Reading a good book
- Joining a support group online
- Drinking hot lemon water
- Cleaning the house
- Taking a bubble bath
- Taking up a hobby that uses your hands (keeping your mind and hands busy) such as knitting or gardening
- Having low-calorie snacks readily available, like fruits or veggies

You will figure out what works for you. When you get an impulse to overeat, think to yourself, What can I do instead of overeating? Sometimes the answer is nothing; you may need to sit through the anxiety until it passes. This may be very challenging to do, but it is also a major step in preventing overeating.

One Reverse Dieter, Melissa, always felt like eating when she had an argument with her husband or one of her children. She had the habit of turning to the kitchen immediately, as she tried to avoid thinking about anything that might have been said in anger. When she felt so mad she wanted to scream, or was offended by an insult, she would overeat. One of her toughest challenges was to sit through that emotion and allow it to pass without eating ice cream, cookies, or whatever sweets she might have on hand. To avoid overeating, she began leaving her kitchen when she would feel an overwhelming emotion come on. "Sometimes I might go and see if there was a movie playing that I wanted to see; other times I might just take a walk around the block. One time it was raining and I couldn't go for a walk, so I grabbed my journal and journaled my way away from overeating."

Reverse Your Work Stress

One Reverse Dieter, Tammy, always seemed to overeat at work or right after work. She loved to eat everything from Chinese to burgers and fries at lunch with her coworkers or by herself during lunch or after work. She might call in an order for dinner before she left the office and pick it up on the way home—usually something unhealthy she was craving. She began troubleshooting this scenario after looking back through her journal. It was then she realized that work was one of her most vulnerable times, when she seemed to eat with the most abandon. Simple awareness that this was when she would most likely overeat helped her come up with other options so she would have alternatives when this particular moment arrived. Here are some things that worked for her:

- She decided what to order for lunch before she was stressed or hungry.
- She brought lunch to work.
- If she didn't have time to fix lunch the night before or the morning of the workday, she made sure there was a frozen low-sodium, low-fat meal in the freezer at work.
- She suggested to the person ordering lunch in the office for everyone that they order from a healthier restaurant or a healthier choice from the menu.
- She picked up something on the way to work from a café (yogurt, apple) to have on hand at her desk.
- She took a walk at lunch for a sandwich, soup, or salad and brought it back to the conference room to eat with coworkers rather than ordering in.
- She had a plan for dinner before she left work in a ball of stress.
- She might decide on her planning day, Sunday, what she'd eat for the rest of the week; or in the morning on the way to work, she would decide what she would eat for lunch and for dinner.

When Tammy made food decisions outside of her work environment, they were usually better. After she'd had time out of her office even for a few minutes, she was able to see more clearly what her impulse was and head it off with a healthier choice. Tammy didn't succeed every time, but three out of five times is a lot better than never changing her eating patterns at all. Hold on to those successes rather than focus on the times you did not succeed. Get used to the feeling of making a better choice.

Tammy realized that she ate in response to the stress and anxiety she felt at work. When she felt the pressure of stress and anxiety coming on, especially when her boss demanded things be done within tight, almost impossible deadlines, she would notice that her reaction was to think about an indulgent lunch or even dinner. She began to look at ways to relieve her stress at work in other ways besides food-related activities.

Tammy started taking a yoga class or another exercise class at lunch and eating a healthy lunch at her desk when she got back to the office, rather than using the whole lunch break to focus on food. By the time she got back to work, the problems she had agonized over seemed a lot more solvable. After discovering the root of her overeating problem, she looked beyond food to where her stress came from and why her job was so stressful. She asked herself if this stressful job was what she wanted in her life long-term. She began applying for other jobs and has recently taken one that is a better fit for her.

While this type of major job change is not always possible for everyone, it is an example of how tracing the real source of stress and anxiety away from food to the root of the problem can help you make changes for the better rather than getting stuck in an overeating cycle that virtually ignores the rest of the issues.

A Note of Caution

Emotional eating has all kinds of sources, from mundane malaise and boredom with your life to traumatic events like the loss of a loved one, a history of having suffered abuse, disease, the loss of a job, or a divorce. The Reverse Diet plan can help you understand your body and remind you to become aware of why you overeat, but it is not a substitute for addressing the problems that motivate detrimental or negative emotions and thoughts that might lead to overeating. If you've suffered a trauma and have issues that need to be sorted out, find a qualified expert who can help you.

Overeating Instead of Facing Reality

Mandy says of her evenings, "When I get home there is usually something I am faced with right away that makes me feel so tired and used up, I don't know what to do. A lot of the time I sit down and have a big meal. Sometimes there are dishes in the sink because the kids didn't do their chores or my two sons have been watching TV instead of doing their homework. After working all day, I feel completely overwhelmed."

When Mandy felt overwhelmed, like many of our clients, she would order pizza or takeout for something she craved, then sit in front of the TV and eat. This helped her ignore whatever had bothered her when she initially got home; she would just block it all out and eat until she was more than full. Then she felt bad about herself for overeating—a more immediate feeling than dealing with the situation at home. Overeating when you're faced with difficult circumstances creates another situation that's tough to deal with—weight gain and dissatisfaction with yourself and your actions. You're sabotaging your body and your self-confidence and avoiding the issues that triggered the bingeing. Rather than solving the problems at hand, you're creating more.

To troubleshoot her behavior, Mandy:

- Made a personal meal plan ready for each night of the week, so that even if she was distraught, she would not have to find a creative solution to dinner—it would already be decided.
- Had prepared meals (cut veggies and meat) in the fridge ready to go into the oven or onto the stove as soon as she got home.
- Rewarded the kids if they did their chores with a once-a-week or once-a-month treat like a movie or a trip to the zoo.
- Ate at the table with her family rather than in front of the TV.
- Sat with her anger, frustration, and disappointment; she took a time out *without overeating* until she was not so overwhelmed.
- Worked on finding real solutions to help resolve some of the

issues that drove her to overeat—like helping the kids with their homework or having them help her prepare dinner.

With all of the successful Reverse Dieters who have specific issues that triggered them to overeat during high-risk times, their success in troubleshooting goes beyond examining the food they are eating, or the all-or-none mind-set. They succeed by becoming aware of their trigger times and figuring out alternatives.

How to Buffer Buffet Habits

Tricia remembers, "Buffets were my favorite. I went to the Giant Panda, a Chinese restaurant, one time. It was all you could eat for $9.95, which included crab legs. I literally sat there for four hours, right hand up! They eventually asked us to leave. My kids were almost falling asleep at the table."

Another Reverse Dieter, Tony, loved buffets. Every time he went to a buffet, he began to overeat. He would put so much on his plate that by the time he was only in the middle of the buffet, not even close to the end, he couldn't fit any more. Tony would then hurriedly eat everything he had on his plate, because he wanted to utilize his chance to go back to the buffet. By the time he left the buffet two to four plates later, he felt stuffed, sick, and guilty.

Tony decided to begin reversing these habits by thinking of ways to get around them. Realistically speaking, Tony wasn't going to avoid buffets for the rest of his life. Instead of dealing with the buffet issue with the all-or-none mind-set by saying he would never go to a buffet again, he came up with alternate plans to overeating. When he would find himself at a buffet, be it a wedding, a party, or going out with friends, he would:

- Make sure he looked carefully at all the food options first before he would begin to fill his plate, rather than just starting at the beginning and taking as much of every kind of food that he wanted.
- Become mindful that a whole plate of food would make him

feel full if he ate slowly, so he began taking his time to choose specific foods he really wanted.

- Eat slowly, cutting food into small pieces, putting his fork down between bites, and sipping water throughout the meal.
- Focus on enjoying *what* he had on his plate rather than *how much* he could fit on his plate, and try to pay attention to the quality of the food instead of the quantity.
- Wait a few minutes before he went up for his second plate so he could allow the food to digest and know how full he really was before he got another helping.
- Sometimes get a smaller plate so his portions would be limited.
- Focus on the conversation instead of the food.

These tips are helpful to anyone who has a tendency to abuse unlimited quantities of food. As any of our successful Reverse Dieters will tell you, the key to changing damaging eating habits is mindful, careful focus on your impulses with food.

REVERSE DIET EXERCISE

Prepare for Your High-Risk Time

Look back over the high-risk times you listed earlier in your journal. For each time, ask yourself the following questions:

- What are a few alternatives to overeating next time you are in that situation?
- What could you do to prevent that situation?
- How can your awareness be heightened *before* you decide to overeat?
- What is the real issue you are trying to mask as you make the decision to overeat or to eat something you know is not healthy?
- How can you address the underlying issue?

Carefully looking over your high-risk times will reveal what is causing the bingeing and what you can do about it. Take note: high-risk times and obstacles are different. For instance, a high-risk time might occur when you are hungry and there is no food available. An obstacle in that scenario might be that you lack the time to prepare healthy food before you are hungry. The solution to this would be to plan in advance. You might carry a snack with you or keep food at your desk (oatmeal, nuts, dried fruit, canned tuna). Overall you should try to think ahead.

Emotional Obstacles

Emotional eating is one of the greatest obstacles for a lot of dieters who have tried all types of diets but still have a negative body image and overeat when they are distraught. To overcome emotional eating, it is helpful to reframe negative thought patterns.

Many of our clients who come to the Reverse Diet have not been able to stay on other diets because they eat as a reaction to an emotional state. If you are one of these people, you eat for mental and emotional placating rather than for physical nourishment. By learning how to reframe some of the thoughts that drive you to food for the wrong reasons, you can begin to examine emotions rather than just eating patterns. Eventually eating and emotions will become separate issues for you, and you can resolve them as they should be—separately.

Many people have an emotional relationship with food. That's not necessarily always bad. Most of us enjoy eating, and we should! It's a great part of life and can be a happy, celebratory activity. Nourishment and enjoyment during the consumption of food should be a positive experience. Habitual overeating and mindless overeating are not the same thing, however. In our society, eating can become a mixed experience involving both comfort and guilt.

Put eating into perspective by realizing why you do it: to nourish and fuel the body and the brain, and on occasion, as part of celebrating holidays and events. As one client, Laura, wrote to us, "Tricia, I don't know how I can ever thank you for leading me to this path of my new lifestyle of eating. I had forgotten how good it feels to eat to get through the day, rather than to get through the day to eat." Laura experienced a pivotal new way to perceive eating.

In this part of the plan, look at the emotions that drive destructive eating habits. Again, it's not unusual to have emotions linked to eating—but it is not good to have them controlling the whole show. Cognizant, mindful eating can take place when you realize you have an emotional trigger, such as boredom, frustration, or anger, that regularly drives you to eat a whole plate of nachos.

One Reverse Dieter, Mary, said of her eating experiences, "When I'm sad or depressed, I go for the sugar and fat, preferably ice cream." She will eat any sugary thing she can find, while sitting on the couch or while working in front of the computer. In some cases, a yearning for a certain food is not only about sugar or content, but about the taste and texture that makes it a particularly good comfort food. Mary likes the smooth and creamy qualities of ice cream. When she's finished overeating, she says, "I feel like a total pig but justify it because I should be allowed to indulge once in a while. The problem occurs when I eat huge amounts and do it for several days at a time." With Mary, it wasn't just the fact that she ate the ice cream, it was the fact that she would eat a whole pint of ice cream at a time, and it was driven by feeling down.

When you realize that your overeating is motivated by emotions, identify which specific emotion is the trigger. For Mary, it is depression. She identifies her depression with a few circumstances: "I'm tired and generally don't want to do much when it's not nice and sunny outside." While we don't encourage you to self-diagnose without seeing a physician, it is a good idea to begin noticing why you feel the way you do. Like Mary, you may get grumpy, sad, or depressed when you don't spend time outside. You may suffer from seasonal affective disorder (SAD), and the solution will not be found in another pint of ice cream.

Alexis, another Reverse Dieter, also works ten-hour days and has an hour commute each way, so she doesn't have a lot of time to be with herself or outdoors. Obviously Alexis can't change the circumstances of the weather or her state after childbirth, but she can begin to cope with her emotions in ways other than eating. She has thought of other activities to engage in when she feels down, besides eating. They include:

- Taking a walk at lunchtime to get some light movement. This may help with fatigue throughout the day so that she is not quite as exhausted at night.
- Eating only at the table (not on the couch).
- Preparing a special portion to indulge in so there is an identifiable limit, like one ice cream cup or one soda pop.
- Investing in lights that make her home brighter in the darkness of winter.

If you eat to resolve emotional issues, you develop cravings. An incredibly important point to understand about yourself is that *when this connection is executed over and over again, it becomes habit.* You begin to associate a certain emotion and a certain food with each other. If you interrupt that habit with a solution, you can begin to reprogram your habits. Try troubleshooting with alternative solutions, and you will be surprised at the outcome and quite proud of yourself. It may take a little creativity on your part, but you can find what works for you.

One theory about cravings is that the less you eat of a particular food you are craving, the less you will crave it. Unfortunately, that craving may not go away forever, but it can diminish with time and have less control over your life and your body.

Another theory states that once a food is *normalized*, meaning there is no stigma attached to eating it and it is incorporated into a healthy, balanced diet, the less likely the food will be overconsumed. A study published in *International Journal of Eating Disorders* in 2005 noted that restrained eaters experienced more food cravings than did unrestrained eaters and were more likely to eat the craved food. So eat what you crave but remember, this is not permission to eat anything and everything you crave in extreme amounts. If you are really craving a particular food, go ahead and have some. Consider that a smaller amount might fulfill the craving. For instance, try a small bit of chocolate instead of a large chocolate bar, try some chocolate sauce drizzled on berries, or take ½ cup of ice cream and put it in a small bowl and enjoy each spoonful instead of eating from the pint (or ½ gallon). Let what you're eating register and satisfy the craving and then move on with your day! Instead of saying to yourself, "No chocolate, no chocolate, no chocolate," reframe that thought and say, "I can eat this chocolate kiss or mini candy bar in small amounts every once in a while."

Reframe Negative Thoughts

Other negative thoughts can stem from negative emotions. As one client, Marcy, said, "I eat when I am lonely, hurt, bored, angry, and filled with self-pity." All of these emotions go hand in hand. Many Reverse Dieters have reported the negative emotions, as listed earlier in the chapter, that trigger their bingeing episodes. Each time you have one of these thoughts, it may become a trigger to overeat.

REVERSE DIET EXERCISE

Reverse Your Negative Thoughts

Take a moment and list the unhealthy, negative thoughts you have regularly. When you have these thoughts again, how can you reframe them to make them more positive? Here are some examples:

- Instead of "I'm fat and disgusting," which often really means "I feel inadequate," ask yourself, "What can I do to feel more adequate?"

- Instead of "I'm ugly," choose a few key things you like about yourself. Have you always liked the fact that you are tall, or your eye or hair color, or your outgoing personality? Replace the negative thought with "I've always had beautiful blue eyes. They are one of my best features," or "I am very empathetic, which is a quality to be valued."

- Instead of "I feel sorry for myself," focus on what you would like to change and how to do it, or consider what you have going for you. For example, "I have a wonderful group of friends and family who love me."

Develop your own personal ways of reframing negative thoughts so that they spur on positive change rather than the repetition of old habits and cravings. Try dealing with the pain without eating. Instead of allowing a negative thought to bring on depression and sadness that will trigger you to overeat or make a poor food choice, recognize that the negative thought gets in the way of your goal. Try reframing those thoughts so that they can motivate you to treat yourself better.

The Reverse Diet is a diet plan geared toward a healthier body, but it's also about making better lifestyle decisions. The power of figuring out your high-risk times and what drives you to overeat can very easily force you to examine other elements in your life that are unhealthy. Emotional eating can stem from poor self-esteem, anger, work, family dynamics, relationships with others, and/or your own negative body image. Once you begin peeling off the layers of your eating habits and patterns and looking closely at which emotions motivate those habits, you may find you'd like to make more changes than just what you weigh.

I love the Reverse Diet! My whole family is doing the plan. When I started the plan, I did it for four months without telling my family, because I was afraid I would fail, and I had failed so many diets in the past. At that time, I weighed 220 pounds. After I started, I was on the Web site every week as Tricia helped me along the way. That was eight months ago, and since then I have lost 70 pounds on the Reverse Diet. When I told my husband I didn't have to pay huge fees every month, just reverse my meals and make sure I was eating Reverse Diet foods, he decided to join the plan. Since then, my husband has lost 35 pounds. I've started my kids on the diet and the whole family is on it now. When we got together for our holiday gathering at my in-laws' home, they were so supportive! They went on and on about how great we all looked. That was my favorite moment.

—Tracy, a successful Reverse Dieter

As you stick with the diet and become better and better at reversing your meals and troubleshooting bad habits, you'll also need to figure out the best way to stay motivated and create a Reverse Diet–friendly environment for yourself. Motivation is key when you're on the Reverse Diet plan. Staying motivated is what helps you have willpower to make good decisions. As Tricia says, "Success is 90 percent from the neck up."

You can also increase your chances of success by identifying environmental obstacles. You'll learn how you can change your environment for the better so that it can assist your weight loss.

Don't Let What Surrounds You Drown You

Your environment can play a crucial role in your ability to resist temptation and old habits. Take a moment to think about what is in your pantry and kitchen. Do you have a lot of things that are not on the Reverse Diet Food List? If so, grab a garbage bag and go to town! Take the dry goods to a food shelter. It doesn't have to go to waste, but that doesn't mean bad foods have to add inches to your waist either!

Check out your pantry and fridge for the following:

- High-calorie, high-sodium dressings
- Highly processed foods such as refined white flour, packaged pastries, cheeses, boxed dinners or cheese crackers.
- High-fat meats, including sausage, bacon, salami, bologna
- Candy
- Processed snack foods (chips, cookies, pop tarts, etc.)
- Frozen items (ice cream, cakes, pastries, processed dinners)

By now you know what is on the Reverse Diet Food List and what is not. Get rid of a food if it's not on the list. You don't have to keep things just because your kids like them. Your kids will benefit from whole foods, too.

Remember, if it's not in your kitchen, it's a lot tougher to eat. Throwing away your old favorite, whether it's ice cream, cookies, or canned cheese, may feel like you're letting go of some old habit you love. To some, it may even feel like letting go of an old friend. You may be sad to see these foods go because they seem safe, but that is not a healthy security.

Raid and purge your pantry when you're feeling upbeat and defiant. Get fired up. Remember, you don't need these foods and your body doesn't need these foods, either. Out of sight, out of mind. Throw out the take-out menus. Getting rid of environmental temptations is the beginning of the end for those late-night snacks!

Are Your Cravings Triggered by Sight or Smell?

As you evaluate your environment, go beyond your kitchen to notice what triggers you to eat unhealthy foods. As you get more and more familiar with what triggers your cravings and what elements create high-risk scenarios, you can also begin to figure out if you are tempted by sight or smell, or both. Some Reverse Dieters find themselves susceptible to smells. For example, just walking by a restaurant or a backyard barbeque and smelling something cooking can make them want to rush out and get a double cheeseburger. Others are motivated to eat by certain things on TV or an ad in a magazine. They might not have wanted a pizza when they began watching TV, but when they see the Dominos commercial, they are overwhelmed with their need to have one. Some people's cravings are stimulated by both sight and smell. Temptations like this can be avoided by getting up and leaving the room when a commercial comes on.

Understanding how you are triggered can help you figure out what to do when you are. That way, you can check your Hunger Scale and see if you are being driven by psychological or physical hunger. Sometimes, simple awareness of your senses can help you act thoughtfully rather than being reactive or impulsive.

For example, if you always walk by Dunkin' Donuts on the way to work and end up getting a couple of doughnuts and coffee loaded with cream and sugar, figure out a way to avoid that high-risk situation. Don't tease or tempt yourself. Take control by choosing another route to work or home so that you are not faced with the temptation of passing a Dunkin' Donuts, a McDonald's, bakeries, or other places where you end up stopping to indulge. This is a good alternative to having to actively fight your habit. Get inventive with changing temptations in your environment—subtle changes in your routine can overcome trigger moments and facilitate big changes in your health.

Reversing Your Kitchen

My cupboards are full of cooking essentials, spices, pastas, brown rice, and containers instead of boxed meals, canned goods, snacks, sugars, and sweets like cookies and Little Debbies.
—Tricia

Make sure you stock your fridge and pantry with some good, healthy alternatives. Just as it matters if you surround yourself with the wrong types of foods, it's important to surround yourself with the right foods. If you fall off the wagon and OD on broccoli or apples—well, it could be worse. If you don't have a tub of ice cream to chow down on when you're having a bad day, that's good. If you must go out and buy something like ice cream, buy an individual portion that has an identifiable start and finish. For example, a Fudgesicle is much better than a pint of ice cream.

Try these suggestions to get started on your new Reverse Diet kitchen:

Pick Foods You Like at the Beginning of Your Plan

Don't just surround yourself with foods you think are supposed to be healthy but you've never actually tried. Filling your kitchen with things you don't like the taste of might just motivate you to run out and get some fast food or quick junk food. In fact, you don't necessarily have to fill your kitchen. If you can't stand beets and radishes and you buy a bunch in a frenzy to eat healthfully, you're setting yourself up for a problem. While it's good to try new foods, do it at a pace that feels comfortable to you. Further into the plan you can experiment with things you've never tried.

Make an Alternative Craving List

Make a list, putting what you usually crave in one column, and making room in the other column for a healthy alternative to the food you crave. For example, Samantha always craves sweet things, like chocolate, cake, and ice cream. On her list she has chocolate and ice cream in the first column, and beside them she has written a few naturally sweet alternatives, like a mango, Tricia's Reverse Cereal, natural peanut or almond butter on a brown rice cake, and yogurt. Often when she goes into the kitchen searching for a piece of chocolate and doesn't know what to eat in its place, she will see her list on the fridge and try an alternative to stop the cravings. When she has cravings, she finds that if she doesn't have a healthy alternative on hand right away, she can fall victim to the same old unhealthy food. Clients who have salt cravings do the same for salty foods. Get creative: if you have a salt craving for chips, you can try cutting veggies like cucumbers or carrots on a diagonal so they look and feel like chips, or have homemade, air-popped popcorn with very light salt or parmesan cheese rather than eating a whole bag of chips.

Throw Away Take-Out Menus

Good-bye Dominos, Chinese Dragon, the local Mexican restaurant, and the burger joint around the corner. Toss the menus in the trash. Have a ceremony if you want. In the long run, these are not convenient and they can take years off your life and put pounds on your behind. If you must have something, eat it carefully and move on; don't keep eating because you think "Oh well, I'm already off my diet."

Don't Listen to Your Kids if They Disagree

So your kids like to go the neighbor's house because they serve fried chicken, Twinkies, and Dr Pepper? They don't want to eat at home because they'd rather die than eat broccoli? They say that their friends won't come over for dinner because you cook "weird" food? Fooey. Just keep experimenting with new recipes. Turkey meat loaf may taste as good as the original meat loaf when they get used to it. And whatever you do, don't feel guilty! Teaching your kids how to have a healthy lifestyle is one of the most wonderful things you can do as a parent. However, if that really doesn't work in your house at all, at least keep snacks—sweet, salty, and otherwise—off the counter. Put them into a drawer or cupboard so that you can reduce impulse nibbling.

Purchase ¼-Cup to 2-Cup Containers for Portion Control

The right sized containers will remind you not to fall into portion distortion. Tricia uses the same size portion containers for freezing meat portions. As she says, "That way there is no guessing when preparing meals. I did this at the beginning so my family wouldn't jump in and eat 'my' food, and I still do it. I know exactly how much cereal mix I am eating because I know the size container it is in." Learning to visualize portions carries over into recognizing how much is enough in restaurants, too.

Freeze Prepared Dinners

You can precook dinner to be ready at a moment's notice. For example, buy vegetables already cut in stir fry pieces, cook them with chicken, then freeze the mix so you can grab it when you're in a hurry. You can add cut-up veggies and chicken to rice in no time flat. It helps to label each container with the contents and the date you froze them.

Reverse Your Restaurant Routine

For many of us, going to restaurants symbolizes indulging. People frequently overeat when they eat out. Very often they allow the restaurant to set the standards for portions and the way a dish is prepared. On the Reverse Diet, many of our clients have learned to change their experiences at restaurants from indulgent, decadent, and damaging to healthful and supportive of their new lifestyles. Following are a few ways to do it:

- **Don't be shy—ask for what you want.** Don't be afraid to ask your server for a healthier dish. Servers are there to serve you, so don't hesitate to ask for any Reverse Diet solution that will make your meal healthier and better for you. More and more people are asking for particular ways they'd like dishes prepared. Servers are used to it these days. You should make your request in a nice, courteous way, and if you feel unsure about yourself, you can tell the server that you're on a special diet and are limiting your sodium and sugar intake. Until she was comfortable and more confident, Tricia even used to fib and say she was allergic, hypersensitive, or diabetic and on a sodium-restricted diet. If the server has to go to ask the kitchen, politely ask that he do so. Your server should not be irritated with you, and if he is, that's his issue and not yours. Chances are, the restaurant will be fine with not dressing a dish in their typical fashion.

- **Have it your way.** Ask to have your dressing, sauce, or gravy on the side. That way you can use your own dressing if you brought it, control the amount of dressing you use, or just eat the food dry or with lemon or vinegar (which isn't a bad thing), or dip your food into the dressing instead of pouring it on.

- **Make smart substitutions and request changes if necessary.** If the menu is unclear, don't be afraid to ask if they serve broiled chicken with vegetables, instead of, say, chicken Parmesan or some other dish with a heavy sauce or high-fat cheese. You might ask that a dish be steamed, baked, or grilled, or broiled rather than fried or sautéed, or for olive oil to be used instead of butter.

- **Plan your meal, even at a restaurant.** As you know by now, planning is a great way to avoid impulse eating. If you're familiar with the restaurant and you know they have a salad or fish and vegetables on the menu, it's helpful to decide before you get there that that is what you'll order. Some Reverse Dieters go a step further and call ahead if they are unfamiliar with the restaurant to have a menu faxed to them—or check online to see if the restaurant has a Web site. If they are going to a business dinner or lunch with a client or the boss, they know ahead of time they will be overwhelmed when looking for a good choice, so they make their selection ahead of time. They are prepared!

- **When ordering a combo, choose one meal** (a meat or fish, not two meals as in surf and turf).

- **To-go boxes are the way to go!** Before you begin your dinner, when it arrives, or even when you order, it can help to remind yourself that you will be taking a portion home for breakfast. As discussed previously, many restaurant portions are huge. Often they can be cut in half. Some Reverse Dieters ask for a to-go box from the very beginning of their meal. They put part of their meal in the box and then just eat what they have left on their plate.

- **Kids' meals aren't just for kids.** Some Reverse Dieters order the kids' portions of meals at dinnertime. That way, they don't have to deal with a large portion immediately. Many restaurants have kids' meals—just make sure they aren't unhealthy. Sometimes there can be dishes like chicken fingers or burgers and fries, in which case, you and your kids should avoid them. You can also ask for an appetizer portion of a main-course entrée. Senior menus are great, too. They are usually smaller than standard entrée sizes, as kid's menus are.

- **Make a meal out of an appetizer.** These days, a lot of restaurants serve appetizers large enough for a meal—especially for a dinner meal on the Reverse Diet. Try looking at the appetizer menu when you're choosing what to order. Often, it can be just enough to get you through until breakfast. Be cautious, though, because often appetizers are the worst offenders in high-fat, low-nutrient food. An unhealthy appetizer can actually add up to more calories and be less filling than an entrée.

Eating out doesn't have to be gluttonous, and you don't have to order high-fat, high-calorie foods. Going out can be enjoyable and healthy if you are attentive to what you order.

Reverse Your Vacations

Preparing for going out is useful on vacation, too. Get creative—you don't have to eat what they give you. Tricia's first vacation on the Reverse Diet plan was bumpy at first, but she was able to keep her eating habits after she took matters in her own hands.

The first time I went on vacation after starting my new way of eating, I was mortified. Until then I was in control of what and how I cooked. Then I went to the beach and there were restaurants everywhere. I had not eaten in a restaurant prior to this event. Even though we had an eat-in kitchen in our vacation unit, I stayed a few miles from where I went to the beach and it was too far to keep running back and forth just to cook my own meals. The first day, I didn't eat. There were no restaurants that served plain meats and veggies—even the potatoes were rolled in salt. I was not in the habit or confident enough just yet to ask for plain meat, veggies, and potatoes. The second day I prepared my own meals myself. I ate my big breakfast, but this time I made two chicken breasts and two baked potatoes and wrapped them in double foil. I placed them in a thermos and put them in a backpack. I took a baggie full of shredded wheat, knowing I could buy OJ at the beach, I packed a plastic bag of fresh broccoli, and I took plastic utensils. I was learning how to prepare for events. Two days of that and I was bored. Not yet ready to stray from the plan, I built up the confidence, went to a restaurant, and asked for plain tuna steak, steamed or cold veggies, and a side of plain pasta, no sauce. To my surprise, I got what I asked for! From that point on, I was not afraid to ask anymore.

Holidays in Reverse

The holidays can also be tough for dieters. People encourage you to eat things that are not good for you—and that certainly are not on the Reverse Diet plan. If Tricia can turn down her grandma, you can say no to anyone!

> Holidays were the hardest for me. My family knew I was eating differently, but how was I going to tell Grandma that the foods she prepared were not healthy things I could eat on my plan? For the first time in twenty-six years, I wasn't eating them. Instead of allowing myself to feel guilty and use it as a license to eat bad foods, I took control of my surroundings. I hosted the first Thanksgiving while on my plan. I let my mom cook the ham; I wasn't eating it anyway. My grandma did the cranberry sauce and desserts, which I wouldn't eat. When it came to the appetizers, potatoes, and sides, they were all mine. Of course, I made it seem that I was going to take all the work on myself and let them relax, when in reality, I was allowing myself control over my environment in order to stay on my plan. I even baked a small chicken breast for me. They loved it all and did not even know tofu was in the potatoes!

One way to incorporate healthy foods into holiday gatherings is to offer to bring a dish, and make something that will be a healthy alternative to some of the more traditional dishes. This way you can eat what you want without calling attention to what you are eating.

Try to creatively find ways to escape bad food choices and you'll find that when January rolls around and everyone's going on a diet because they aren't happy with the state of their body, you'll be on a healthy, stabilized eating plan.

Motivate to Lose the Weight

I began the Reverse Diet four months ago and have lost 27 pounds. Usually I have good days, but sometimes, I do have bad days. When I have a rough day, I go to my e-mail and read the e-mail posts of other Reverse Dieters on the Web site and how wonderfully they are doing with the program. Whenever people post things that are positive, it helps me so much. It's like an extended family. Most of the people on the Web site know what it's like to have a bad day, where you might have eaten too much of the wrong thing, and they also know how to make you feel better about it and help you get back on the program.

I have failed at losing for so many years—I feel that I lost my youth to being overweight—but I pray that I will live out the rest of my life slimmer and healthier, and I can tell I'm already on my way. Thank you for sharing this weight-loss program with us, and thank you for your support. It means so much to have a chance to get rid of my weight, feel better about myself, and get on with my life.

—Margaret, a successful Reverse Dieter

Figuring out how you can get motivated and stay motivated is a big part of losing weight and staying on the Reverse Diet plan. You're already motivated because you're reading this book. That's the easy part. The trick is to stay motivated past the initial phase of losing weight.

Your body will process food the way it's supposed to if you give yourself the correct food and amount at the right time of the day. Success in losing weight is not just about what you put in your body and what you don't, it's also about your mental commitment to your body and a healthier lifestyle.

The Reverse Diet Club:
Motivation by Support

Many Reverse Dieters have found that support makes a huge differ-ence. Online is a great place to get questions answered and find motivation from others who are going through the same thing you are. This can help keep you focused on your goal. The Reverse Diet Club is an online club for members of the Reverse Diet plan. Not only is there a forum for you to voice victories, news, concerns, and questions, but it also provides another type of structure. With encouragement, accountability, and a goal to reach every week, the online club adds a special dimension to your experience on the Reverse Diet.

Members love being a part of a group that they can relate to. The support groups meet each week. There are no scales—just fellowship, motivation, networking, and answered questions. Many of our mem-bers like to read online community posts as often as every day to help keep their own goals in focus. Tricia frequently answers questions online or posts new recipes. She loves to hear from anyone on the plan and can be contacted at membership@reversedietsolution.com.

Marcia, a Reverse Dieter, says, "I have followed it to a T, joined the support group, and am feeling so awesome. . . . I am full of energy and my self-esteem is soaring. I cannot wait for a new day to start to see how well I have done." As many of the members have found, shar-ing your success can be a rewarding part of weight loss, especially if it helps others.

A Reverse Diet Friend

If you can, find someone to do the Reverse Diet with. If you share your goal with someone else and check in regularly, often you will feel more accountable and supported. Sometimes dieting can be lonely, espe-cially when no one else around you is doing it. Checking in via e-mail, by phone, or in person once a day, once a week, or once a month with a Reverse Diet friend can be a great way to keep your momentum.

You can also reveal your cravings and weakness to your Reverse Diet friend so they are aware and can touch base with you regularly. Consoling each other when you overeat or sharing recipes is a great way to feel like you have support twenty-four/seven. Brainstorm ways to avoid overeating. Your Reverse Diet friend can be your husband, your mom, your daughter, a neighborhood friend, or someone online in the Reverse Diet Club. Chances are, if you investigate and find the right friend, you'll end up checking in regularly. And you'll have a buddy to celebrate with as you drop your pounds.

When we asked one of our original Reverse Diet members what helped her, she said, "Get a buddy, write a journal. Talk, talk, talk; it is so hard to do it by yourself. We need someone who understands exactly what we are going through. Someone who will not judge the amount of food we eat."

You need someone who will not judge you, but who will support you. That's what you should look for in a Reverse Diet friend.

Reverse Diet Goal Reminders

Staying motivated is something that needs to be constantly reinvented. If you set a goal and make it, the toughest part can be after you reach that goal. Continuing or maintaining to lose weight can be hard, especially when you're used to rewarding yourself with food (and not usually the healthy kind!). Tricia used to reward herself with overeating anytime something good happened. "If I passed a test— burger and fries, here I come!"

As we've discussed, you should pick realistic goals. Some of your goals don't have to do with weight. It's a good idea to reevaluate your goals throughout the plan and make them visible to you in your daily routine. You can post your goals throughout your house, car, or office so that they remind you to stay on your plan. Here are some of the places our clients often post them:

- On the refrigerator
- On the bathroom mirror

- As a screensaver on the computer
- On the center console of the car
- On the desk area at work
- On the pantry
- In their PDAs

You can post more than just goal weights. Many of our clients post messages like:

- I will eat only when hungry.
- I will stop eating when I am full.
- I will plan my meals ahead of time.
- I am strong enough to resist temptation.

One client, Susan, said "Visual stimulation and reminders of how good I'm doing help me resist pigging out." These reminders can help Reverse Dieters acknowledge how they've done so far and how far they have to go. This can be as simple as just writing a positive note to yourself and posting it somewhere you will see it often.

You may want to try to regularly reinvent motivational goals. If you do, pick a day at least every month (maybe on the first) to revisit the reasons you are motivated to stay on the diet. You can do this more often if you like, once a week or even once a day in the beginning. Whatever day you choose, that day you should journal about why you are motivated and what differences becoming healthier is making and will make in your life. Hold these issues in the forefront of your mind.

What Motivates *You*?

What motivates you may be different from what motivates other people. Do you have a particular event that you'd like to look your best for? A class reunion or wedding is often something that sparks motivation to lose weight. Anything that motivates you is good, but it's also important to realize that if it is an event, the toughest part will be staying on track after that event.

While it's fine to allow yourself to lose some weight for a special event, we advise that you don't hang all your weight-loss hopes on that one date. Instead, if you plan all along to lose weight for the long term, and specifically a certain amount by a particular time, the special event can serve as a benchmark point rather than a be-all, end-all moment. That way, you don't have the immediate loss of a central goal after that date passes. Short-term or process goals, known as action steps, are what you do to get to your goal weight, or long-term goal. An example of a process goal is "I am going to plan my meals for tomorrow, today." That goal will help you achieve your goal weight.

When choosing goals to motivate yourself with, try to have short- *and* long-term goals, and make the distinction between them. Here are some examples of long-term outcome goals:

- Looking good this summer in a bathing suit or shorts
- Losing weight for a wedding
- Losing weight for my family's vacation
- Losing weight so I can wear a pair of jeans I used to fit into
- Breathing more easily
- Having better health as I age
- Being able to be more active throughout life
- Feeling better in clothes
- Sleeping better
- Walking more easily
- Feeling more confident

Short-Term and Long-Term Goals

You'll recognize some of these long-term goals as the realistic goals discussed in chapter 1 that you can maintain in a healthy lifestyle. Working toward good, solid long-term objectives makes it easier to maintain dedication to a new eating plan and to develop eating habits for life that will contribute toward a longer and better life.

REVERSE DIET EXERCISE

Assess Your Goals

Remember to regularly assess what your short- and long-term goals are and how to keep them fresh. Try revisiting them in your journal a few times a week.

Short-Term Pats on the Back

Short-term goals are the action steps (process goals), and the long-term goals are the results of these action steps. It is helpful to find things to reward yourself with that replace food rewards. There will be immeasurable rewards as you begin to feel better about yourself, but it's a good idea to shift the focus off food for practical rewards, since many dieters have used food in the past to reward themselves. If you lose a few pounds, feel good about yourself, and haven't fallen off the wagon all that often, treat yourself to a special reward weekly or monthly:

- A massage or some other spa treatment.
- Tickets to a favorite sporting or musical event.
- A new outfit or piece of clothing in your new size—(maybe a new belt, scarf, shoes, hat, or pajamas).
- A new cooking utensil.
- A new bubble bath or bath oil.
- Money in your dream vacation fund.
- A new CD.
- An hour to yourself to take a walk or be with friends.

You know what will work for you. Put notes on your calendar for each week or every other week so you know what's coming up. A note like "concert" or "new book" can outline what you'll get if you stick to your plan. Pick a day, perhaps each Saturday, when you can have a small scheduled reward, or every other weekend if you've been on the plan for a while. Figure out something that makes you smile or feel good and put it in your line of vision.

Scheduling rewards is a great way to give yourself a pat on the back. You deserve it, and the more you let yourself know that you deserve to be treated well and to treat yourself well with other rewards besides food, the quicker you'll be able to break your old habits. Think outside the box!

Breakfast, a Time for Motivation!

Make breakfast a time of day you look forward to that anchors you in your busy day. Tricia says, "Breakfast has become my family's dinner in more ways than just food choices and portion sizes. Our family sits down for breakfast and we discuss the day before us and what we hope to accomplish. Everyone is home for breakfast, but dinner often feels like shift work, with each member of the family off on extracurricular activities like sports, music, or dance classes. Breakfast time gives you smiling faces, great expectations of the day, and a time to set goals. Dinner is quick with no hassles and leaves more time to do chores, relax, or go to the park or gym—no more slaving over a hot stove for hours of cooking, eating, and cleaning up when you'd rather be relaxing!"

Use breakfast as a refuge and an event to begin your day in the right way, whether you have a family or just want some quiet time for yourself. Allow it to help set the mood for the rest of your day.

Reverse Diet Tips

- Just cleaning out your kitchen, house, or pantry once won't do it. You have to keep on constant alert that things don't creep in. Does your husband buy junk food and bring it home? Around the holidays, do you find more cookies and candy at work or sent as gifts to your home? There's nothing wrong with regifting a huge tin of cookies if staying on your plan is more important.

- Record your short- and long-term goals in your journal and check them off accordingly. Remember to give yourself a nonfood reward and a pat on the back when you deserve it.

- Try to reinvent what motivates you occasionally. Make sure you're paying attention to how much weight you are losing; making a note of actions you take to improve more than your health can help you feel good enough to continue even through a plateau.

- Remember that you can ask for whatever you need at restaurants, you're not putting anyone out.

- Remotivate yourself one day at a time and you will prevail in high-risk moments.

PART TWO

The Reverse Diet Bridge Phase

6

The Reverse Diet Bridge Food List and Meal Plans

When I first began the Reverse Diet, I had 25 pounds I wanted to lose that I couldn't seem to get off no matter what I tried. I had tried low-carb diets that didn't work. It was especially hard for me because I have type 2 diabetes and I'm fifty-four years old. I decided to try this diet, but I showed it to my doctor first. Because of my diabetes, he tweaked it a little so that it suited my blood sugar requirements. In three months, I lost those 25 pounds and have kept the weight off for a year! I use the Web site all the time and have a lot of friends on the support group. Seeing people I haven't seen in a while is such a joy, because of the compliments I get. They are so proud of me!

—Marissa, a successful Reverse Dieter

The Reverse Diet Bridge

The second phase of the Reverse Diet is the Reverse Diet Bridge. This is the phase in which you have reached your goal weight, you feel great, and you want to begin reintroducing foods that are not on the Reverse Diet Food List. Whereas the first phase can last anywhere from two months to a year, the Bridge Phase may last about three months. This can be a scary period for some because they may have finally reached their goal weight and don't want to jeopardize their success.

In this chapter, you will learn how to bring foods that you like back into the diet without sacrificing your new body. You will learn how to cross the Reverse Bridge from the world of the Reverse Diet Food List to a newfound freedom with foods you used to feel out of control around or used to abuse and overeat. Along with your new freedom will come the necessity to eat them in appropriate, mindful portions.

You Look and Feel Fantastic—Now What?

You reached your goal weight and now you want to transition into eating food that isn't on the Reverse Diet Food List. Your confidence has returned! You're a new person and feel like a million bucks. You have redefined yourself in the process of shedding weight and habits that did not support your goals, while keeping all that you liked about yourself in perspective. And it was worth it. You've been in a world of special Reverse Diet foods and mind and body training. As you step out into the rest of the world, you may be faced with a lot of foods and situations you have worked hard to avoid. Be mindful that you are better prepared and are more aware now.

There is a way to eat the foods you used to eat—white bread, white pasta, chips, fatty meats, and desserts—without gaining the weight back. Though some Reverse Dieters lose interest in those foods for good, some of our clients want to reincorporate them and are scared or apprehensive at this stage. Tricia was worried that she would fail and gain back the weight she lost if she took chances with her old favorite foods like nachos. She was afraid that once she took a bite, she might revert to her old habits and lose control. A lot of Reverse Dieters feel the same way once they hit their goal weight. They celebrate, and then look around and wonder how they will transition without gaining all the weight back. With the new skills and the mindful attention you have worked hard to attain, you can do this! As Tricia figured out and as Heidi teaches her clients, you can introduce those foods back into your life simply with smaller portions—one day at a time, one meal at a time.

Your new eating options are not all-or-none—avoid that dreaded mind-set! By now we hope you have learned you can eat until you are almost full and then eat again later when you are hungry. You will find you can eat a mindful portion of cheese, chocolate cake, chicken wings, or a not-so-healthy food of your choice and know you don't have to eat a lot of it because you can always eat it again if you choose to. It's just a food choice. The food choices we make regularly determine the health and adequacy of our diets. Remember, everyday foods—the foods that are the foundation of your new healthy eating habits on the Reverse Diet—are different from occasional foods that sometimes fit your moods or social situation and may not fit the diet. It never has to be all one way or another. People who are successful at weight loss and maintaining it stay constant and don't indulge in wild abandon every holiday or vacation.

Your Fire Is Burning

Just as you must carefully put logs on a fire so it will continue to burn, you must carefully choose the correct portions of foods at the right times to fuel your metabolism but not give it too many calories to burn at a time. Too much or too little fuel puts the fire out. With too little, the fire dwindles, with too much, it is smothered—but just enough and the fire burns bright and constant. Finding the balance between how much food and when to eat will help you stay at your current weight. While you can eat a cheeseburger and fries occasionally, you must limit your portions. Your body will burn it off if you are mindful of how you eat.

At your goal weight you will probably not be as hungry as you were in the beginning of the weight-loss phase. Keep this in mind as you prepare yourself mentally for old foods, without the old feelings or habits that you had before the Reverse Diet. You've been losing weight on the weight-loss phase, so it's only natural to fear that change will bring weight back. It doesn't have to, if it's done properly.

Once you achieve your goal weight, you can increase your calories a bit because you are maintaining; you are in a calorie balance. When losing weight, you are in a calorie deficit; when gaining, you are in a calorie overload.

Adding Some Foods but Not All

Even though you're allowed to add some different foods back into your diet, you don't need to add *all* unhealthy foods back into your diet. Try to avoid the feast-or-famine cycle that so many get caught up in. Here is a quick list to give you an idea of the different foods that can be cautiously integrated back into your diet:

The Reverse Diet Food List (Bridge Phase)
Foods you can add back in moderation (read labels for sodium and fat content):

Yellow cheeses (infrequently)

Fat-free hot dogs (watch the sodium)

Whole wheat multigrain breads

Low-sodium, low-fat turkey bacon

Lean beef or pork in moderation

Sugar-free preserves and jellies

Sugar-free, salt-free peanut butter

Barbecue sauce

Worcestershire sauce

Decaf coffee

Light beer

White wine and red wine (in moderation)

White liquors (tequila, rum, vodka, etc. in moderation)

No-sugar-added juices (fresh fruit is still a better choice)

Low-sodium snacks, chips, crackers, unsalted pretzels

Here is a brief list of some foods to avoid integrating into your diet, as they do not contribute to a healthy lifestyle if eaten on a daily basis:

Reverse Diet No-No's (Bridge Phase)

Abundant salt

Sugar (or items with added sugar)

Lunch meats from the deli (often these have too much sodium, but Healthy Choice meats are allowed)

Artificially sweetened juices and drinks

Prepackaged dinners, frozen or boxed, that are high in sodium and processed meats

Fatty meats (any)

Canned vegetables (unless they are low-sodium)

Canned fruits (unless they are in unsweetened natural fruit juice)

Any food that you associate with overeating

Keep these lists in mind as you choose what to integrate into your diet. Remember, take it slowly until you've got a handle on balancing your hunger and your body's needs with the foods you want to eat.

Eating New Foods with Caution

Even though you're allowed to eat some processed foods in the Reverse Diet Bridge Phase, if you want to maintain your weight, you have to maintain your portions. By now, you should have a lot of practice in paying attention to portion size. When you begin introducing new foods into the diet you have established for yourself, you need to take baby steps. You've entered the unprocessed food world as a new person, with a new body and a new metabolism. The need for awareness about portions especially applies to processed foods.

In the first phase, you slowly adjusted your ideas about processed foods by seeing how they affected your body. Now you have to make the choice:

- Whether or not you will integrate them into your diet.
- How you will deal with your old eating habits when they inevitably return, even if the impulses are weaker now than they were.
- How much of these foods you will eat a time.

You are probably better at visualizing portions than before the diet began. Here are some things to keep in mind about portions if you begin experimenting with fatty and/or processed foods not found on the Reverse Diet Food List:

- Start with a portion of the particular food about the size of your fist until you know what portion size your body can handle without gaining weight.
- If you're eating pizza, keep it small—one slice, not three—and round out the meal with a salad and/or fruit.
- Try one scoop of ice cream instead of two or three.
- Remember, if you exceed your portion size, you will gain weight and you will have more work to do losing it.
- When you are thinking about exceeding a small portion, ask yourself—is it worth completely eliminating this food from my diet again or can I enjoy limited quantities?

Try to fully evaluate the repercussions of eating huge portions of unhealthy, processed foods. Be mindful of what you are really doing to yourself and your body. You've been down that road before. Ask yourself, did it work for you? Sometimes all it takes is a good, thoughtful moment before you start on your second slice of cake. If you take that opportunity and move away from the plate of food or table, consider what strategies or internal dialogue you have practiced that you can call on during this moment. If you do decide to pig out, consider the results:

- You will move closer to participating in the weight-gain cycle that you worked so hard to escape.
- Your body will not feel as good as it did when you ate moderate portions of food; after overeating you may feel uncomfortably full.
- The negative thoughts and feelings that accompanied your earlier state may return.
- Your lean, mean, fat-burning machine will get bogged down—overeating unhealthy foods is the equivalent of throwing wet logs on a fire or putting water in your car's gas tank.

- Your energy will decrease.
- You may feel self-defeated.

You know that all of these things happen when you overeat. You knew it before you became a successful participant in the Reverse Diet. What is different when you're in the Reverse Diet Bridge phase? You now know how it feels to:

- Have a better quality of life when you are healthy.
- Eat appropriate serving sizes and stop when or before you are full.
- Breathe more easily when you walk across a parking lot.
- Feel better with an improved body image.

REVERSE DIET EXERCISE

Take Stock of the Benefits

Grab your journal and take a moment. What have your personal results throughout the weight-loss phase given you? Are they similar to the list above?

Use these new experiences to avoid overeating. Use them to be more mindful of how and what you eat. Now you've got something to lose besides weight—a healthy body and a better life!

Reverse Diet Bridge Menu Plans

Here are two weeks of menus of what your meals might look like in the Reverse Diet Bridge Phase, taken from Tricia's journal. Keep in mind that the recipes for the Reverse Diet dishes can be found in chapter 9 and that the recipes make more than one serving—make sure you're controlling your portions.

WEEK 1

Day 1

Breakfast

Reverse Diet Breakfast Wrap

Glass of skim milk

Hot lemon water

Snack

Dried apricots

1 cup of nonfat yogurt

Lunch

Reverse Diet Pasta Salad

Tilapia filet with garlic butter sauce

Snack

Orange

Dinner

Tofu stir fry with green beans, onions, and peppers

1 cup of brown rice

Hot lemon water

Day 2

Breakfast

Reverse Diet Meat Loaf

Glass of skim milk

Hot lemon water

Snack

Reverse Diet Apple Smoothie

Lunch

Reverse Diet Stuffed Tuna Tofu Tomatoes

1 cup of mixed greens with 2 tablespoons of fat-free dressing

Hot lemon water

Dinner

Mixed fruit salad and low-fat yogurt

1 ounce of almonds

Day 3

Breakfast

> 1 turkey sausage
>
> 3 to 5 small whole wheat pancakes and 2 tablespoons of sugar-free syrup
>
> Glass of skim milk
>
> Glass of orange juice

Snack

> Reverse Diet Baked Apple

Lunch

> Reverse Diet Scallops with Linguini in Tomato and Basil Sauce
>
> Roasted red peppers
>
> Hot lemon water

Dinner

> Reverse Diet Apple and Tofu Dip with Assorted Fruit Platter

Day 4

Breakfast

> Reverse Diet Meat Loaf
>
> Reverse Diet Scalloped Potatoes
>
> ½ cup of corn
>
> Hot lemon water

Snack

> Reverse Diet Stuffed Mushrooms with Crabmeat

Lunch

> 1 cup of Reverse Diet Clam Chowder
>
> Slice of whole wheat toast
>
> 1 glass of grapefruit juice
>
> Hot lemon water
>
> 1 apple

Dinner

Tropical fruit and tofu smoothie

Day 5

Breakfast

2 scrambled egg whites with tomatoes and mushrooms

Cup of cubed watermelon and cantaloupe

Hot lemon water

Snack

Reverse Diet Rice Cake Pizza

Lunch

Reverse Diet Sloppy Toms topped with lettuce, onions, and tomatoes

1 serving of Reverse Diet Coleslaw

Hot lemon water

Dinner

Orange and peach smoothie

½ cup of shredded wheat

Day 6

Breakfast

2 eggs (done your way)

2 slices of low-sodium bacon

Slice of whole wheat toast with low-sodium, low-fat butter substitute

Glass of skim milk

Snack

Banana on a whole wheat bun topped with 2 tablespoons of low-fat, low-sodium peanut butter

Hot lemon water

Lunch

> Reverse Diet Southern Shrimp Creole
>
> Sliced kiwi
>
> Hot lemon water

Dinner

> Mandarin orange salad with almonds over baby spinach with 2 tablespoons of low-calorie, low-fat dressing

Day 7

Breakfast

> Western omelet
>
> 1 cup of potatoes fried in extra-virgin olive oil and garlic
>
> Glass of orange juice
>
> Hot lemon water

Snack

> Reverse Diet Salmon Roly-Polies

Lunch

> Fruit cup with nonfat yogurt
>
> Sliced chicken breast
>
> Reverse Diet Barbecue Sauce for dipping
>
> Carrots and celery sticks

Dinner

> Peanut butter and jelly sandwich (low-fat, low-sodium, sugar-free) on whole wheat toast
>
> Glass of skim milk

WEEK 2

Day 1

Breakfast

> 4 ounces of lean pork chop

½ cup of potatoes fried in extra-virgin olive oil

½ cup of Brussels sprouts

Snack

Sugar-free gelatin

1 cup of mixed berries

Lunch

Whole wheat pasta

Reverse Diet Quick Spaghetti Sauce

Steamed spinach

2 tablespoons of Parmesan cheese

Dinner

Cooked oatmeal with sliced apple and raisins

1 cup of nonfat fruit yogurt

Day 2

Breakfast

6 ounces of swordfish steak using Reverse Diet Caribbean Jerk
Sauce

Reverse Diet Twice-Stuffed Potato

½ cup of baby lima beans

Hot lemon water

Snack

½ cup of low-fat, low-sugar ice cream topped with 1 cup of
strawberries

Lunch

Reverse Diet Veggie Soup

Grilled cheese sandwich on whole wheat made with low-fat
cheese

1 ounce of mozzarella cheese

Hot lemon water

Dinner

Melon ball salad with 1 cup of frozen yogurt

Day 3

Breakfast

Reverse Diet Piggyback Enchiladas

Corn and black bean mix

½ cup of fried rice with cayenne pepper

Hot lemon water

Snack

½ cup of low-fat cottage cheese with ½ cup of peaches

Lunch

Shrimp cocktail

2 cups of spinach salad with 2 tablespoons of low-fat
dressing

Glass of no-sugar-added cranberry juice

Dinner

Reverse Diet Mac and Cheese Bake

Reverse Diet Stuffed Celery

Hot lemon water

Day 4

Breakfast

Reverse Diet Clucky Chicken Pot Pie

Hot lemon water

Glass of orange juice

Snack

½ cup of Succotash with 2 tablespoons of low-fat sour cream

Lunch

Reverse Diet Pasta Salad

Grilled pork kabob with squash, peppers, onions, and cherry
tomatoes brushed with oil and garlic mix

Hot lemon water

Dinner

    Creamy broccoli soup

    Mixed fruit smoothie

Day 5

Breakfast

    Reverse Diet Shrimp a la Queen

    Reverse Diet Veggie Soup

    Hot lemon water

Snack

    Strawberry smoothie

Lunch

    Grilled veggie platter (eggplant, tomatoes, purple onions, red, green, and yellow peppers) over tossed greens

Dinner

    2 hard-boiled eggs

    1 cup of low-fat cottage cheese

    Glass of orange juice

    Hot lemon water

Day 6

Breakfast

    4 ounces of lean top sirloin marinated in Reverse Diet Honey Dijon Pizzazz Marinade

    Slice of garlic whole wheat toast

    ½ cup of cauliflower with low-fat cheese sauce

    Hot lemon water

    Glass of orange juice

Snack

    Reverse Diet Fried Zucchini

    ½ cup of low-fat cottage cheese

Lunch

    Reverse Diet South of the Border Fiesta on Cornbread

    Hot lemon water

Dinner

    Reverse Diet Spinach Dip with assorted veggies

    2 plums

Day 7

Breakfast

    Reverse Diet Egg Bake

    Hot lemon water

    Sliced strawberries

Snack

    Baked low-sodium tortillas

    Reverse Diet Sassy Salsa

    Low-fat sour cream

Lunch

    6 ounces of sliced turkey breast

    1 cup of oven-baked french fries

    Reverse Diet Cranberry Sauce

    Hot lemon water

Dinner

    Reverse Diet Sweet Potato Pie

    Glass of skim milk

    1 apple

Tricia also added whole wheat toast and cheese sticks to the menu. Tricia was able to eat these foods because she made sure she ate moderate to small portions. Again, you may not be as hungry as you found yourself before in the weight-loss phase. If you are not hungry for the food or snack, do not eat it.

Appreciate Your Reversed Taste Buds

So you used to love to eat chocolate cake and used to crave it all day long? When you ate it, maybe you couldn't get enough. Nothing could satisfy like that cake!

One of our clients, Cindy, reached her goal weight of 140 pounds, down from 211. During the plan, she had not strayed very far from the Reverse Diet Food List. Now, only a couple of weeks after reaching her goal weight, her daughter wants to have a chocolate cake at her birthday party. She orders the cake, decorates it herself at home, and all the while is wondering, will she dare to have a piece at the party? For months now, she hasn't given in to her chocolate cake cravings more than a few times. The guests arrive, the birthday song is sung, her daughter blows out the candles, and she is handed a piece of cake. She gingerly takes a bite and is hit with a surprise—ewww! It's so sugary—too sweet, actually. It tastes like pure sugar. The icing itself seems to stick to the roof of her mouth and she ends up scraping some of it off the cake so she can eat the rest of the piece. I used to like this? she asks herself.

This is a common story. After eating healthy whole foods for a prolonged period of time, our taste buds adjust to the natural sugars in fruit and we crave the refined sugars of processed foods less. Cindy found the same extreme was true when she had french fries with salt on top. The fries seemed too salty and did not taste as good as she remembered.

Another client, Andrew, had the same experience with the premium ice cream Haagen-Dazs. He ate some after avoiding it for a few months and found that, compared to frozen yogurt, it tasted too rich, thick, and sweet.

The reversal of your taste buds after you have been on the plan for a while will help you in the Reverse Diet Bridge Phase. This is not to say that you won't like your old favorite foods again, but they will taste a little foreign when you begin eating them after they have been absent from your diet for a while. This change will help you regulate those old cravings.

Just because you have reached your goal weight and are able to eat the old favorites again doesn't mean you have to. Tricia still hasn't gone back to eating sweet or processed foods regularly. She eats them only on special occasions or occasionally. She prefers to fix foods the way she did in her early days of the Reverse Diet, with exceptions here and there. As she says, "I have had only half a piece of pizza since 1999. I do not even desire the old unhealthy foods and I don't feel deprived. I have a whole new world of foods—unhealthy foods do not control my life." Tricia's success has led her to detach herself from processed foods that at one time she used to live for. She still likes certain foods and has her weaknesses, but she has found greater control over her cravings after developing a whole new way of eating.

You don't have to avoid processed foods altogether. Heidi loves pizza and usually has one slice a week. Her portion size usually depends on whether or not the pizza crust is thick or thin and how much meat or cheese is on it. She has learned how to still have pizza, a favorite food, while maintaining a mindful balanced Reverse Diet. For her, inevitably there is a day when she is running late and can't make it home to cook, or she's out at dinnertime and pizza is the easy, convenient choice. She saves pizza for those times, and when she does have it she doesn't get meat toppings, but she primarily has vegetables on top. You can personalize your long-term diet in a similar way. Pizza is just cheese, bread, and tomato sauce—basically healthy ingredients when not overdone.

You've had a taste of reaching your goal. If you have faith in yourself, your success, and what you have accomplished, you will have strength to stop when it's enough and be able to prevent overeating.

REVERSE DIET EXERCISE

Take a Reverse Moment

The trick to executing portion control is to give yourself that essential moment before you begin eating. This is the moment in which you tap into an unconscious relationship with food and evaluate it from an objective perspective. Whether it is an emotional or environmental obstacle that has triggered this moment, you might be on the brink of allowing it to kick your bingeing into high gear.

For example, you have had a long day, everything seems to be overwhelming, and finally, you order a pizza with several meat toppings and extra cheese. You haven't had one in so long. It arrives and you think, "Oh what the heck, I deserve this." All you can think about is how that pizza will taste and that you can't get enough.

It is in that moment that you must stop and ask yourself, "Is it really worth it?" Then look at how far you've come and say to yourself, No, *I'm* worth it.

The response to "I'm tired and overwhelmed and hungry" is "I need to relax, breathe, and eat one slice." Eating a whole pie will not make you feel better or less overwhelmed. You know this because you've done that before. This is a Reverse Moment. These are powerful moments when you realize that you are stronger than your old eating habits. You can have one or two slices and put the rest in the freezer or even the garbage. Or in that moment you may decide you don't want to order the pizza. Don't order something you don't want to eat much of, especially when you know it's a large portion, until you are confident you can eat only what is appropriate for you. If you find that you cannot just have one slice, then you need to take that moment and take that breath before you order the pizza next time. Go to a restaurant where you can order by the slice or make a choice other than pizza.

Heidi has learned from her experience with clients that some who overeat often believe in the moment of overeating that they "deserve" that particular food. Maybe it is because they have had a rough day or maybe it's in celebration of something. Either way, they use it as a justification. When she probed deeper, she began seeing that the idea of deserving really meant that they were lacking support elsewhere. They weren't getting something they needed—a close relationship, help with household chores, understanding about the workload at work, or a similar problem. It came down to a frustration they were feeling that translated to them feeling it was okay to overindulge or overeat.

During the weight-loss phase, you were not purposely facing temptations. You might have fallen off the wagon here and there, but you avoided those old trigger foods if you could. Now you are facing tempting, unhealthy foods in an effort to move on with your life and are maybe eating them at times. To get to the point where you can cope with these temptations, you have to build a bridge, one plank at a time. One small appropriate portion at a time, you will build your bridge to a normal diet that works for your body.

REVERSE DIET EXERCISE

Take a Deep Breath

The next time you are ready for a meal or snack, practice taking a careful, deep breath before you begin eating. Try to make it last at least ten seconds. Close your eyes if you like. It might be helpful to go into another room where there is no food. If you are with a group of people, go to the rest room and take the breath there if it helps you concentrate. This gives you a chance to reflect on mindful eating and listen to your conscious awareness. Figure out what works for you. This doesn't have to be right before eating something "bad" for you. It's a good idea to practice before eating healthfully, too, so that when you begin to integrate other foods into your diet, you're ready with your breathing technique.

In this moment of silence you take for yourself, carefully consider why you are eating and how much you would like to eat. While you are taking that moment, it's helpful to consider two things:

- Set a portion goal. How much are you planning to eat before you begin? Without a plan, you are more likely to overeat. The plan doesn't have to be rigid—it is more like a mindful thought because you will also be paying attention to your hungry and full signals.

- Remind yourself that *you eat to live, rather than live to eat.*

You'll be surprised how calm, cool, and collected you feel after that breath.

The Reverse Buster

During the Reverse Diet Bridge Phase, it's not unusual for your body weight to vary on average from 5 to 8 pounds. Everyone is different; some may not vacillate at all whereas others will. If and when the scale goes up, you can shift into high gear and switch for a day or two to the Reverse Buster. Tricia uses the Reverse Buster when she overeats or feels off track. One Superbowl Sunday she pigged out on nachos, wings, and wine all day. As she said:

> I did not worry about it too much because I stayed on the plan throughout the week before. The Superbowl was all day long, though, and then for the next couple of days I was off the plan. I went to put on a pair of jeans I had on the week before and they were snug. I got on the scale and committed to being serious. I had to get on the Reverse Buster because my system was out of whack. I stuck to the Reverse Buster and now I am back to eating what I want in moderation. I won't be so inclined to pile the nachos on anytime soon.

While Heidi often tells Reverse Dieters that they can't actually gain weight in one day—often a difference on the scale can be seen in water gain—you still might feel shaken, guilty, or off track after bingeing. As she tells her clients, if you get back on your program immediately, you will not suffer long-term weight gain.

When you fall off the wagon, just determine what you need to do to get back to the process of weight loss. You can make an effort to change your behavior, avoid binges, and work on making a better choice in the future. We do *not* recommend doing the Reverse Buster for more than three days. This is a low-calorie quick fix and cannot healthfully sustain you for more than a short period of time. Here is a specific diet to follow if you binge.

Tricia's Reverse Buster

Breakfast

    Hot lemon water with ginger

    ½ cup of cereal mix with ½ cup orange juice

    4-ounce chicken breast with 1 tablespoon of extra-virgin olive oil

    ½ cup chopped celery

Lunch

    Hot lemon water

    4 ounces of fish with 1 tablespoon of olive oil

    2 ounces of tofu

    ½ cup of spinach

Dinner

    Hot lemon water

    2 ounces of tofu

    ½ cup of cereal mix and ½ cup orange juice

    ½ sliced cucumber

The results are amazing. Not only will you feel healthier than ever, you will feel empowered to continue on the plan. It's hard work, but it has a dramatic, immediate payoff.

Coping with Overeating in the Bridge Phase

One Reverse Dieter, Marlene, reached her goal weight of 120, having lost 60 pounds. She had been hard at work sticking to the plan and had begun to supplement it with exercise (more about exercise in the next chapter). She felt good and was getting compliments every time she turned around. It was amazing what an effect this had on her self-esteem. For her anniversary with her husband, two weeks after she had reached her goal weight, they decided to go out to dinner to an Italian restaurant she used to go to before she began the Reverse Diet. She always used to eat large pasta and veal dinners there late at night, at least once a week. Old memories of lots of tasty food came back as she ordered what used to be "her usual." As they waited for the food to come, she drank red wine and freely ate the bread at the table, as she hadn't done in months. When the food came she ate as much as she could—almost all of the spaghetti and a breaded veal dish in a cream sauce. The portion was nearly triple what she was now used to eating, especially at dinnertime.

After eating, Marlene felt the old familiar feeling of too much food in her stomach. She said of the experience, "I felt awful! I immediately had the thought, 'Now, why couldn't I just eat a small amount and take the rest home?'" When she e-mailed Tricia for a solution on how to rectify the situation after the huge dinner she had eaten, she got these tips:

- **Give yourself a break—cautiously.** Overeating happens, and you've been conscientious for a long time. *Importantly, you don't want to jeopardize your success by allowing it to justify carelessness.* Remember, eating more refined carbs and processed foods may make you crave them even more. Even though you should avoid punishing yourself in any way, that doesn't necessarily entail allowing yourself to eat whatever you want.

- **Stay away from the scale for three days.** Don't freak out and jump on the scale the next morning. Give your body some time to process everything. Allow it to level out. Work on eating foods on the Reverse Diet Food List.

- **Remember, this happens to everyone.** Marlene learned that bingeing was not worth that feeling. The important thing to take away from experiences like Marlene's is that even though you can't beat yourself up for overeating, you also have to take it as a warning that you need to be more mindful. Know your limits and remember your goals. By beating yourself up and giving into a guilty feeling, you are feeding a negative overeating cycle. Move on, get back to basic action steps in the Reverse Diet plan, and don't add insult to injury. Many people overeat more when feeling bad about overeating. Instead, remember the behavior and attitude that got you to your goal. Forgive yourself and move on.

As Tricia said about the bridge phase,

When I was in the Reverse Bridge stage, it took me months before I was able to eat anything not on the plan. I did not feel comfortable eating other foods, and when I began to, I took baby steps. I had experienced too many times before that when I began eating other foods, I thought to myself, It's okay to splurge; I just lost all of this weight. I did that many times before and lost control, gaining all the weight back and more. This time I had worked too hard and I was not willing and didn't want to repeat the struggle, so I really paid attention to everything I ate. I noticed I was not as hungry so I did not eat as much as I did while losing—I continued the big breakfast, medium lunch, and small dinner routine, just using smaller portion sizes. It worked and I stabilized my weight.

Tricia and many other dieters have learned to take it slow. Maintaining your pattern of eating and not consuming too many foods that aren't on the list in the beginning of the Bridge Phase is the key to learning how much of what foods you can eat.

Journaling through the Reverse Bridge

A huge motivational tool for Tricia was her journal. Keep your journal regularly throughout this second phase. When you hit a spike in your weight, look back and see what eating trends might have caused it. Watch out for your trigger moments and high-risk times. They could redevelop and you might have new triggers and high-risk times different from the first phase.

Journaling is a great way to stay motivated. Tricia used her journal for food lists and also to check in with herself daily. As she put it, "Holding myself accountable was really good for me. I would write down daily goals in the morning and check my accomplishments off at night. It was incredible to see all those checks. I did it every day." She chose different goals that were easy to achieve and reminded her of her quality of life. They might remind her to check in with her family or to enjoy her time to herself. They gave her other things to focus on besides just staying on the Reverse Diet plan. Her journal underlined the fact that she had other pieces of pie in her life besides just her weight or diet. Here are some goals from Tricia's journal:

I will laugh at least five times today.

I will hug my kids two times each today.

I will stay away from cigarettes today.

I will take one half hour for me (walking, meditating, or doing something besides eating) today.

I will call my grandma today.

I will call my mom today.

I will make someone feel better today.

I will continue to follow my Reverse Diet plan today.

I'm going to read a chapter from a book today.

She says, "These were realistic goals to achieve. I knew this and created my list accordingly. They seem simple. At first I would see this long list. But it's fun to see all the items checked every day. I still do it!"

This is a great example of Tricia personalizing what motivates her and makes her feel good about herself. What works for you? Maybe it's similar to what Tricia is doing, although your list may be very different, and that's okay.

Tracy, another Reverse Dieter, said on her list:

I'm going to read before bedtime.

I'm going to carve out time to play outside with my children.

I won't answer the phone when I'm with my children.

I'll sit at the table and eat without any distractions or the TV on.

I will not wear my sweats all day.

I'll write a quick note to a friend I've been out of touch with.

I will continue to follow my plan today.

Other dieters work toward goals like signing up for volunteer work or just getting to work on time. Perhaps you have another way to check in with yourself on a daily basis so you can remember why you're doing what you're doing on the Reverse Diet plan. Be creative when you tackle these daily or weekly check-ins with yourself. It pays in many creative small ways to stay motivated—this ends up helping the big picture.

Start Looking for Your Purple Dress

As you cautiously reintroduce foods back into your life, don't forget to enjoy your new self. For everyone, this will be different. For Tricia, it was finding a dress that would symbolize her celebration and success all in one. She says:

> It was New Year's Eve, December 31, 1999. I had been on my plan for many months and was now a size 9! To celebrate, I was going to go out on the town and buy a new dress. It would be my first official outing. Few had seen me this whole time and only remembered what I used to look like. I had no money to go to the mall, but there was a discount store in my town. This was last-minute on the thirty-first, but I was determined to find the one that would match my great mood. The dress that caught my eye that day was a beautiful shimmering purple floor-length gown. It had spaghetti straps and was snug to the hips and lightly fell to the floor. I wore my hair up, bought matching shoes—even my shoe size went down as I lost weight!

I went to a club in my hometown. Everyone I had known before was going to be there. As I walked through the double door entrance, the most extraordinary feeling overcame me. It was like a Hollywood movie scene. So many of my old friends were in awe and could not believe it was me. Some of these people had never known me to be thin. The compliments came in double doses, not only for the weight loss but for how I carried myself and how my confidence had grown. It was truly a night to remember. I still own the dress and even though it is too big now, I pull it out and wear it for those occasions where I want to feel really special! My husband smiles as I'm pinning it up or tucking it in and he even helps sometimes. He knows what that dress means to me.

Recognizing your achievement can happen in all sorts of ways. One client, Ryan, who lost 80 pounds, says his "purple dress" is new camping gear, and he goes on hikes and camps all the time now, as he never did before. Before the Reverse Diet, he had a tough time catching his breath from the parking lot to his office. Going camping is a new addition to his life that helps him remember how far he has come.

Another Reverse Dieter, Rachael, who lost 60 pounds, has taken up tennis. She plays three times a week and can hardly believe there was a time when she was afraid to wear a sleeveless shirt and skirt and play the same game that she used to love as a little girl. "That tennis racquet has come to symbolize my new abilities and my new life I've discovered. I love getting on that court with confidence instead of the self-conscious feelings I used to have."

Now that you are on the bridge that will take you from reversing your body to reversing your life, take a moment to think about making a new addition to your life.

Reverse Diet Bridge Tips

- When introducing new foods into the second phase, remember to exercise portion control.

- Before eating a new addition to your diet, take a breath and decide how much you're going to eat of that particular food. Give yourself permission to stop and have more later that day or another day.

- Notice how the new, less healthy foods affect how you feel and your energy level. Do you feel good when you're finished eating them? How does that feeling compare to eating a well-balanced meal with whole, unprocessed foods?

7

The Reverse Diet Accelerated: Building Lean Muscle and More

A few months ago, I had a checkup and the doctor told me I was one clogged artery away from a stroke. After hearing Tricia's weight-loss stories on TV, I decided to try the Reverse Diet and see if I could get myself healthy. When I began the Reverse Diet, I followed the diet and began to exercise more than I had in years. I even began feeling so good after I exercised that I started doing it almost every day. I went back to the doctor six months later and my LDL, or bad cholesterol, was down 40 percent. The Reverse Diet turned my life around.

—Jerry, a successful Reverse Dieter

Perhaps you've been doing well on the Reverse Diet plan, so well that you want to know how to accelerate your experience. This chapter will help you do that. Whether you're eating right, following the weight-loss phase, the bridge phase, or the third phase—the maintenance phase—you may want to expand on your new Reverse lifestyle with a few other things that can complement the program, some of which can speed up your weight loss. We'll talk about those and also go over some tips that can help you make meal preparations easier, experiment with certain foods that many Reverse Dieters have come to love, and discover other ways you can enrich your experience with the Reverse Diet plan.

Reverse Your Perspective on Exercise

For many people who have struggled with poor body image, who have spent years hiding their body instead of celebrating it, the idea of working out may even seem a joke. One of Heidi's clients said, "My idea of exercise is pushing away from the table." In reality, the joy and positive body awareness that physical fitness can bring are so great, once you get in the groove, you won't want to stop.

Engaging in regular physical activity is one great predictor of being able to maintain weight loss. According to the National Registry of Weight Control, exercise ranks as one of five action steps that people who have lost 30 pounds or more follow regularly.

It's true that Tricia did lose quite a bit of weight without vigorous or regular exercise. While she did walk often, she did not join a gym, get a personal trainer, or adopt a fitness regimen that would significantly contribute to her weight loss. Science tells us that the best bet for maintaining weight loss is to include regular physical fitness. Exercise is a healthy element of a well-rounded lifestyle. In any of the three phases, you should exercise.

Exercise Is One Way to Build Lean Mass

As Heidi tells all of her clients, exercise can help burn calories and maintain lean mass. Lean mass, which is muscle, burns calories even when at rest. Fat weight is storage weight. That is why you do not have to "feed" your fat weight—fat storage does not use energy; it stores potential energy. In contrast, muscle uses energy by burning calories. Some individuals who have become sedentary and overweight even have fat throughout their muscles. Repeated weight cycling or yo-yo dieting without exercise may leave your body fatter each time weight is put back on. When you lose weight without exercise, you are likely to lose both fat and muscle tissue. When you put weight back on without exercising, you put mostly fat back on. Weight cycling adds to the challenge of weight loss by adding fat and reducing metabolically active lean mass. Losing weight through diet alone without exercise can be done—it is just healthier and easier in the long run to incorporate basic physical activities to support your long-term goals.

If you have been a yo-yo dieter, it might be an especially good idea to consider weight training, which will help keep you toned. The less lean mass, or muscle, you have, the fewer calories you can burn. Exercise that helps to build or maintain lean mass is especially important as we diet and as we age.

There are some terrific benefits to exercise that will improve your long- and short-term quality of life. Some of these include:

- Easier breathing
- Better psychological well-being
- Better general fitness and better ability to walk, run, and be physically active

Exercise reduces the risk of:

- Premature death
- High cholesterol
- Colon cancer and breast cancer
- Diabetes
- Heart disease
- Anxiety
- Depression
- High blood pressure
- Bone density loss issues (especially important during weight loss)

Exercise helps you maintain or lose body weight or body fat and assists in the development of healthy muscles, bones, and joints. How could you not want to exercise after you look at the facts? Habit. The habit of not exercising, just like bad eating habits, can be hard to change.

Jump for Joy

We recognize that exercise can be intimidating at first if you have not been physically active in years (or ever). Here are a few tips to help you get started:

Choose Something You Like

Find a physical activity you enjoy. Walking the dog? Biking? Hiking in the woods? Does music motivate you? Get an iPod or try an exercise class. Don't begin with an advanced-step aerobics class if you know in advance you're uncoordinated and don't like to remember routines. Don't take a spin biking class if you can't stand biking. Find something you enjoy. You'd be amazed at the different fitness classes. Some gyms even have cinema rooms where you can do cardio and watch a movie! Try a video in your home. Do some research and think about what appeals to you. Did you take a martial arts class when you were young and love it? Maybe try a kickboxing class. Does this all seem like too much? Try yoga or Pilates. Start slowly and comfortably and go from there. Figure out something that works for you.

Work on Strength Training to Help with Building Lean Mass (Cardio Plus!)

You don't have to do heavy weight lifting. You can do various forms of resistance exercise. Using body weight, or exercise balls, machines, light weights, or exercise bands—these are all acceptable methods. Keep in mind that working on strength training with cardio supports muscles, ligaments, and tendons, and helps prepare you for long-term body maintenance. If you want to start with weights instead of cardio, that's perfectly fine, as long as you take your first step.

Exercise in an Environment You Like

If you get an unpleasant taste in your mouth when you think about going to the gym, think about your alternatives. There are plenty of them, and they don't cost money like a gym membership. Some people really enjoy walking outside. Try it and see how it works for you. A brisk walking regimen gets you into fresh air and sunshine, big mood boosters in and of themselves. If you live in a cold climate, you can still exercise outside. In any outdoor store, you can find garments made from new fabrics that allow for exercise outside in cold weather.

If you decide to join a gym, do some research and make sure it's the right one for you. For example, if you're a woman uncomfortable working out around men, there are alternatives—all-female gyms like Curves. Try to find an atmosphere that feels comfortable when you go to work out.

- **Set achievable goals.** Just as Reverse Dieters are urged to set realistic goals for their weight loss, you should do the same with your beginning exercise regimen. Setting yourself up for goals that will be tough to achieve is sabotaging your attempt to exercise. Use goals to overcome your personal challenges.

  - Do you know exactly what your challenges are? Take a moment with your journal to explore what they might be. If you're intimidated by the whole concept, think carefully about why. Having trouble breathing when taking the stairs? Cardio is the answer. Is it difficult just to carry your own grocery bags? Lift weights to get stronger. Physical fitness is functional! Don't know how or what to do? Read on, we will make some suggestions.

  - Is it tough to find time to work out? If so, set aside time on your calendar and work toward keeping your workout dates. Work with your obstacles, not against them. For example, if you don't feel you can work out because of your kids, take them with you on a walk, go to a park, or take them on a mild hike. Many facilities offer child care.

- Do you need an event to motivate you? If so, choose a race (5K, swimming, biking, etc.) or event that is suited to your abilities and far enough in the future so that you have time to get in shape. If you're not a veteran runner, don't plan to run a half marathon in the first month you begin working out.

- Do you need to feel accountable to someone else? A personal trainer might be what you need to get you started. Additionally, a personal trainer can help educate you and give you the skills and knowledge you can use to feel comfortable working out on your own. A good trainer will help you get started at the correct level of exercise for you and help you build your strength and stamina in appropriate increments. There is some wonderful and inexpensive online guidance. Heidi recommends www.plusoneactive .com as a great resource for qualified trainers. Another option is an exercise partner akin to the Reverse Diet friend. Partner up for trips to the gym, long walks, runs, or bike rides, or try an online fitness coach.

- **Don't go overboard.** When you haven't been exercising regularly for a long time, don't set yourself up to exercise six days a week for two weeks—unless you're an atypical case, you likely will burn out. Begin with a moderate schedule, like three times a week, as little as ten to twenty minutes a day during lunchtime or after work, and see how it goes.

Build physical activity into your schedule so it becomes a habit!

Branch Out with Food

Another way to accelerate your healthy lifestyle is to try foods you haven't tried. Broadening the foods you typically choose can help increase your healthy eating choices and stave off boredom.

Tricia earned the name of Tofu Princess when she broadcast all the benefits of tofu on the local news one day. It is her favorite main ingredient in her new Reverse lifestyle. In an interview about her success on the Reverse Diet, she shared her newfound love of tofu with listeners and days later, local stores found they were sold out of tofu and still getting lots of requests for it.

Why tofu? If you're not sure what tofu is, it's the curd left over after processing soybeans. Soybeans are great—in the pod they are easy to eat as finger food. The beans can be processed into various food forms and used in place of milk, cheese, or meat.

Tofu has an attractive consistency and is bland, which means it's able to take on the flavor of whatever seasoning it is cooked with. If blended with the right ingredients, tofu has a creamy texture and can serve in place of sour cream or mayonnaise in a variety of recipes, including salad dressings, spreads, shakes, sandwiches, and desserts.

Often used as a meat substitute, soy is a high-protein plant food. It can be eaten alone or in any dish you would normally prepare. Working plant-based proteins like tofu into your diet can help you avoid proteins that have more fat, such as fatty cuts of meat.

Soy contains phytonutrients and may offer protective health benefits, including:

- Reducing the risk of heart disease
- Helping protect against various cancers
- Fighting menopausal symptoms
- Fighting osteoporosis
- Assisting in weight loss

Tricia has had guests to her house and made a meal for them that included soy, and most people didn't even know it was added to a recipe. Quite a few Reverse Dieters have found soy to be a welcome new discovery after beginning the diet. Daphne, who had overwhelming cravings for sweets, said, "Ever since I started eating tofu, I've been craving it! Wow, I never thought I'd say, 'I crave tofu!' I'm really loving the stir fry that I make with my extra-firm tofu and chopped veggies. It's soooooooooo good!" While we can't promise that your sweet cravings will disappear, we can say that you might find soy a new favorite food if you try it. You can substitute tofu in any of the protein recipes in the back; just use tofu instead of chicken or turkey. There are even tofu smoothies!

Reverse Diet Caution

Women with a history of estrogen-positive breast cancer should check with their doctor before adding a significant amount of soy to their diet.

Accelerated Accessories

As you begin preparing your own meals more, you'll start figuring out what speeds up the prep work and you'll figure out your own style of cooking that suits your tastes. Tricia has also been called the Nuke Queen, since she uses her microwave so much when she's cooking and reheating meals. On road trips Tricia has even stopped at gas stations, convenience stores, and grocery stores and used their microwaves. "I have never been refused!" Heidi loves traditional oven and stove-top cooking. She doesn't even own a microwave. The chart below will give you a good comparison of approximate cooking and heating times using a microwave and an oven. (The minutes in this list are approximate and will vary per microwave or oven.)

Food	Microwave	Oven/Stove top
Fish	2–5 minutes	5 minutes per inch of density
Chicken breast	3–7 minutes	10–20 minutes
Baked potato	2–6 minutes	50 minutes
Soups	4–10 minutes	5–10 minutes
Veggies	1½ minutes	steam, in time it takes water to boil
Soufflé	2½ minutes	25 minutes
Eggs	1–1½ minutes	3 minutes

Oven temperatures may vary. You can find recipes for both oven and microwavable dishes with specific cooking instructions on cooking Web sites such as www.epicurious.com. You'll find what works with your lifestyle and personal preferences, just as Tricia and Heidi did. It's helpful to experiment and try new things.

Blenders can be very time-efficient tools for the Reverse Diet plan. As Tricia likes to say, "In a pinch hit the switch!" She uses a blender for smoothies, fruit juices, soups, sauces, condiments, and vegetable meals on the go.

A great blended drink doesn't have to come from a recipe. Create your own using your favorite ingredients! This is a perfect way to have an easy-to-carry snack or meal in the car when you're in a hurry, without worrying about the hassles of eating. As you sip a healthy, blended drink, remember that just because you're drinking and not eating, you still are consuming calories that count as a meal or a snack.

High-Octane Reverse Foods

As you become more familiar with the Reverse Diet Food List, explore some new types of foods. Some have great benefits, others are just foods you might come to love. If you have never tasted half of what is on the Reverse Diet Food List, try one new vegetable a week. Each provides unique and powerful nutrients that can help keep the immune system strong, delay the effects of aging, maintain a healthy blood pressure, improve eye health, delay diseases such as macular degeneration, and reduce the risk of heart disease and cancer.

- **Orange juice** provides a healthy dose of vitamin C for antioxidant protection and immune support. OJ also provides folate and potassium, two nutrients important for heart health. Potassium helps with the body's fluid regulation and to counterbalance the effects of sodium in the diet. Plus, an orange has over 170 different phytochemicals and more than 60 flavonoids, many of which are shown to have anti-inflammatory, antitumor, and blood-clot-inhibiting properties.

- **Shredded wheat** made from 100 percent whole grain wheat is a good source of vitamins B_1, B_2, B_3, E, folic acid, calcium, phosphorus, zinc, copper, iron, and fiber. Whole grains reduce the risk of metabolic syndrome, and women who eat whole grains tend to weigh less.

- **Oatmeal** is a good source of soluble fiber, which can help decrease cholesterol levels, provide cardioprotective benefits, and help maintain blood sugar levels in people with diabetes. Oatmeal also contains zinc, copper, and selenium.

- **Broccoli,** a cruciferous vegetable, contains phytochemicals sulforaphane and indoles that provide significant anticancer effects. Consumption of broccoli is shown to contribute to significant reduction in heart disease risk as well.

- **Spinach** contains flavonoids, which function as antioxidants and as anticancer agents, and carotenoids, which are found to fight prostate cancer and protect against age-related macular degeneration and cataracts. Spinach is also a good source of vitamins K, C, and A, folate, and magnesium.

- **Beans** are high in soluble fiber, which promotes healthy digestion and slows blood sugar response and can help lower cholesterol. Beans also provide B vitamins to help release energy food and iron, which is important for the oxygen-carrying component of blood. Beans also provide protein.

- **Eggs** provide a good source of high-quality protein. Studies now show that eggs do not significantly affect cholesterol levels in most individuals. Eggs also provide vitamins A, E, B_{12}, D, riboflavin, folate, selenium, zinc, lutein, and zeaxanthins.

- **Yogurt** is a very good source of calcium, phosphorous, riboflavin, iodine, B_{12}, pantothenic acid, zinc, potassium, protein, and molybdenum. The friendly bacteria, *Lactobacillus bulgaricus* and *Streptococcus thermophilus*, help to maintain gut health and may prevent vaginal yeast infections in women. Studies also link lower body fat to consumption of calcium-rich foods. Adequate low-fat dairy consumption can help with bone health.

- **Tomatoes** contain lycopene, which is protective against colorectal, prostate, breast, endometrial, lung, and pancreatic cancers. Tomatoes are an excellent source of vitamin C and vitamin A, and a very good source of potassium and vitamin K, and a good source of niacin, vitamin B_6, and folate. Interestingly, lycopene is more bioavailable after cooking than before.

- **Mushrooms**, including the common button mushroom, are shown to have anticancer properties. Crimini mushrooms are an excellent source for a variety of B complex vitamins, selenium, riboflavin, pantothenic acid, copper, niacin, potassium, and phosphorous. Shiitake mushrooms are shown to lower cholesterol levels in animal studies.

- **Garlic**, regularly consumed, lowers blood pressure, triglycerides, and LDL cholesterol (the "bad" form) while increasing HDL cholesterol (the "good" form). Compounds in garlic also reduce inflammation. Plus, garlic is an excellent source of manganese, a very good source of vitamin B_6, and vitamin C, and a good source of selenium.

- **Blueberries** are loaded with antioxidants, which are known to help fight cancer and may lower cholesterol. Blueberries can help relieve both diarrhea and constipation. The tannins found in blueberries can reduce inflammation in the digestive system.

- **Grapes** that are purple in color contain the flavonoids quercetin and resveratrol, which appear to decrease the risk of heart disease.

- **Chili peppers** contain capsaicin, which helps reduce inflammation and may work as a pain reliever. Red chili peppers like cayenne are shown to reduce cholesterol and triglyceride levels and increase the body's ability to dissolve fibrin, a substance that is integral to blood clot formation.

- **Nuts** provide a wide variety of benefits. Walnuts are an excellent source of omega-3 essential fatty acids; a quarter cup provides 90.8 percent of the daily value for these essential fats. Omega-3s provide cardiovascular protection, promote better cognitive function, and provide anti-inflammatory benefits. Almonds are high in monounsaturated fats, which are associated with reduced risk of heart disease. A quarter-cup serving is rich in vitamin E, magnesium, and potassium, and even includes calcium. Cashews are lower in fat than most nuts, provide healthful monounsaturated fats, and are a good source of copper, magnesium, zinc, and biotin. Nuts provide fiber and protein.

- **Salmon** is low in calories and saturated fat, yet high in protein and omega-3 essential fatty acids. As little as one serving of this "brain food" a week may significantly lower your risk for Alzheimer's disease. Regular consumption may reduce your risk of arthritis and depression.

- **Cod** is an excellent source of low-calorie protein. It is a good source of omega-3 fatty acids. It also provides vitamins B_{12} and B_6, which are needed to keep homocysteine levels low and can reduce the risk of heart disease.

- **Extra-virgin olive oil** is rich in monounsaturated fat. People who regularly use olive oil especially in place of other fats have much lower rates of heart disease, atherosclerosis, diabetes, colon cancer, and asthma.

- **Onions**, regularly consumed, are shown to lower high cholesterol levels and high blood pressure and reduce the risk of heart attack or stroke. Several anti-inflammatory agents are found in onions that may be helpful in reducing pain and swelling.

- **Cucumbers** are composed mostly of water; they also contain vitamin C and caffeic acid, both of which help soothe skin irritations and reduce swelling. Cucumbers consumed with their skins are also rich in fiber.

- **Celery** is rich in potassium and sodium, helping to rid the body of excess fluid—they are natural diuretics. Celery also contains vitamin C, which can support immune function, and phalides, which may help lower cholesterol.

- **Parsley** is legendary for its ability to help keep breath fresh. Parsley is also a source of vitamin C, beta-carotene, and folic acid.

- **Strawberries** are a rich source of phenols, primarily anthocyanins and ellagitannins, which makes them cardioprotective and anticancer; they also offer anti-inflammatory benefits and are high in fiber and vitamin C.

- **Romaine lettuce** is extremely low in calories and is dense with nutrients, such as beta-carotene, folate, vitamin C, manganese, and chromium. Romaine lettuce is also a good source of dietary fiber.

- **Iceberg lettuce**, although low in nutrients compared to other lettuces and greens, makes an excellent wrap instead of a tortilla, bun, or bread.

Put some of these foods on your grocery list if you haven't already. Trying new foods is part of learning a new lifestyle. Eventually you'll have your own list of favorite foods that you like as much as those old processed foods you thought you couldn't live without.

Another way to expand your selection of cooking ingredients is to try growing herbs or vegetables. If you don't have a backyard garden, you can do this on a terrace or windowsill with pots. As Tricia says, "I grow a lot of my own herbs and tomatoes. It is fun to watch them grow and they make me proud. I grew these myself! Even if you live in the city, you can grow them in a window all year long."

Savvy Reverse Substitutions

Learning new ways to make foods you like is a great way to transform your habits, satisfy your cravings, and still eat in a way that is enjoyable. Each successful Reverse Dieter develops her or his own favorite recipes or tweaks old recipes so they eat healthful ingredients that support their goals. No need to feel guilty after eating. Below are a few of Tricia's favorites. You will find specifics in the Reverse Diet recipe chapter on how much to use, how long to cook, and so on, but this will give you an idea of how to transform old staple meals from your old eating habits into healthy Reverse Diet meals. Remember to exercise portion control.

- **Lasagna.** Substitute whole wheat pasta, low-fat ricotta cheese, and homemade tomato sauce or low-sodium prepared sauce. Add veggies such as eggplant, crumpled tofu mixed with low-fat ricotta cheese, ground turkey, or plain tofu as your main ingredients. Top with part-skim mozzarella cheese.

- **Pizza.** Use whole wheat flour for the dough and homemade sauce or low-sodium prepared sauce. Add tons of veggies, crumpled tofu, diced chicken, and ground turkey. Top with part-skim mozzarella cheese. You can also use whole wheat pita bread for the crust. This is great for phase 2. Sprinkle with Parmesan. Some creative ideas include pineapple and chicken pizza, pizza loaded with fresh tomatoes, broccoli and tofu pizza, and spinach, mushroom, and ground turkey pizza.

- **Beef burgers.** Try lean ground turkey instead of beef. Be sure to buy the ground meats that do not include the skin. Ground turkey or ground chicken breast may be your best choice for lower fat. Other alternatives include venison, buffalo, veggie or soy, salmon, or very lean beef. Meat labeled "select" is a leaner choice of meat than the "choice" grade.

- **Steak.** Choose lean cuts of meat such as top round, round tip, sirloin, filet, and flank. Cut away all visible fat. Use low-fat cooking methods such as roasting or grilling, which allow fat to drain away. For an alternative to meat try portabello mushrooms, which have a steaklike flavor. They can be marinated or grilled.

- **Spaghetti.** Use whole wheat pasta and homemade or low-sodium prepared tomato sauce. Spaghetti squash is a fun substitute too, because it has a similar texture, but it's a healthy vegetable. Most important with pasta is to control your portion size. Bulk up ½ cup to 1 cup of pasta with lots of veggies, fish, chicken, or low-fat cheese.

- **Ice cream.** Use fat-free, sugar-free ice cream with less than 90 milligrams of sodium per serving. You can also try low-fat or fat-free frozen yogurt. Be cautious of the tempting toppings, which add lots of fat and calories. Try freezing fat-free or low-fat yogurt for another creamy delicious treat, or even puréed fruit, which, when frozen, makes a wonderful natural sorbet.

- **Sugar.** Use sugar substitutes or very small amounts of the real thing. Cinnamon, nutmeg, ginger, or vanilla can enhance the sweetness of foods without your having to add additional sugar. Experiment with these spices.

- **Salt.** Try a salt substitute. Fresh herbs and spices such as rosemary, thyme, oregano, garlic, onion powder (not onion salt), and lemon juice help to enhance the natural flavors in foods.

- **Milkshakes.** Use skim milk instead of regular milk. Add tofu, fat-free/sugar-free yogurt, and fresh or frozen fruits along with ice for different varieties.

In baking and recipes you can easily substitute these alternatives to reduce the fat without reducing the flavor:

Cheese	Try low-fat cheese
Whole milk	Use 1% or skim milk
Eggs	2 egg whites equal 1 egg
Oil	Reduce the oil by half and add applesauce or puréed prunes (for baking)
Butter	Use low-fat margarine that contains zero trans fats

Flour   Use whole wheat flour

Sugar substitutes for cooking include:

- **Sucralose (Splenda):** You can cook with Splenda, but it does not brown or caramelize the way sugar does.
- **Aspartame (Equal or Nutrasweet):** It can't be used for cooking (it breaks down with heat), but you can sprinkle it on top after cooking or use in cold dishes.
- **Saccharin (Sweet 'N Low):** It can be used for cooking but it does not brown as well as sugar and baked goods are often dry and tough textured.
- **Sugar alcohols (sorbitol, maltitol, erythritol, xylitol):** They can be used for cooking.

Once you get the hang of substituting old, unhealthy ingredients with new alternatives, you'll be able to tweak any recipe. Following is an example.

Original unhealthy recipe:

Beef Tacos

¼ pound high-fat ground beef

taco seasoning in a packet

2 taco shells

½ diced tomato

¼ chopped onion

shredded lettuce

¼ cup sour cream

½ cup shredded cheddar cheese

¼ cup diced black olives

Brown beef and mix with taco seasoning. Place taco shells in oven wrapped in foil and bake at 325 degrees for 10 to 15 minutes. Layer taco with beef, tomato, onion, lettuce, sour cream, shredded cheese, and olives.

Healthy recipe with Reverse Diet substitutes:

Reverse Diet Turkey Tacos

¼ pound low-fat ground turkey

½ diced jalapeño pepper

¼ diced green pepper

¼ teaspoon chili powder

¼ teaspoon black pepper

¼ teaspoon thyme

1 teaspoon minced garlic

½ teaspoon Parmesan cheese

2 baked taco shells (no salt)

½ chopped tomato

½ chopped onion

½ cup shredded lettuce

¼ cup fat-free sour cream

handful of black olives

½ cup shredded part-skim mozzarella cheese

Brown turkey and mix in seasonings with jalapeño pepper, green pepper, Parmesan cheese, and garlic. Bake taco shells in oven at 325 degrees for 10 to 15 minutes. Layer meat mixture, tomatoes, onion, lettuce, and sour cream, and add olives and shredded cheese.

As you can see, it's easy to enjoy the same dishes by substituting ingredients. Pretty soon, you'll think the Reverse Diet version tastes a lot better, too!

When I heard about the Reverse Diet last year, I was eighteen years old, and I felt a little overweight. I lived with my parents and was about to begin community college the next summer. I saw Tricia on TV and decided to try the Reverse Diet to get myself in shape and ready for college. The problem was that my family wasn't used to eating food like the meals on the Reverse Diet. My mother and father are from Mexico and they prepare traditional Mexican foods that aren't exactly low in fat or cholesterol. My mother prepared all our food at home–I didn't know how to cook. I didn't want to offend my mother by telling her I couldn't eat her cooking, so I told my mom that I wanted to learn how to cook and help her prepare meals. That way, when I began to introduce Reverse Diet recipes, it wouldn't seem as if I was just telling her how to cook differently, but that I would be helping. Eventually, after cooking a few Reverse Diet meals and discussing the concept of the diet with her, she was on board to help me. We figured out new ways to turn our traditional meals into Reverse Diet meals. The whole family began eating better, and I lost 25 pounds! My mom, father, and brother lost between 10 and 25 pounds each, too.

—Maria, a successful Reverse Dieter

Stay on the Reverse Bridge for as Long as You Need

The bridge phase can last as long as you need it to. Typically it is about three months. That doesn't mean it won't take a lot less or a lot more time to adjust to eating moderate amounts of other foods that are not on the Reverse Diet Food List. It may take a few months of encountering different situations to experiment, learn how to include foods back in your diet, and feel centered when being mindful is still an effort for you. Sometimes going back to the basics of the weight-loss (first phase) principles can serve as a security blanket. Some Reverse Dieters switch back and forth between phase one and phase two until they feel ready for the final phase, the maintenance phase. Others are ready to follow the Reverse Diet Maintenance Phase for life.

See what works for you!

Reverse Diet Bridge Tips

- Try a little exercise and see how it feels. Find something you like that doesn't intimidate you. This can begin with just a walk around the neighborhood.

- Try putting on some music to make the exercise more enjoyable. Start small and slowly, depending on your fitness level, with five, seven, ten, or fifteen minutes.

- Try foods you have never had before. Working soy protein into your diet is a great way to find alternate types of protein. If soy is already an old favorite of yours, try another healthy food you've never eaten, like eggplant or mango.

- Work on converting some of your old favorite recipes you have been avoiding during the weight-loss phase into Reverse versions. Get creative and experiment with ingredients. Have fun!

PART THREE

The Reverse Diet Maintenance Phase

8

The Reverse Diet
for Life

*Before I began the Reverse Diet, the type of clothing I would buy
and wear was mostly large shirts from men's department stores.
I liked them because they were big and loose and would hide my
body. With the Reverse Diet, I've gone from 190 pounds to 155
pounds. Now I'm wearing shirts and pants that show off my figure instead of trying to hide it, and I feel feminine! I also feel
more confident with my career and I'm making other changes
in my life. I feel younger too. I sometimes get a little embarrassed about the compliments I have been getting, but I secretly
enjoy every one of them.*

—Jill, a successful Reverse Dieter

When I entered into the Reverse for Life stage, I was not worried about my weight any more. I was confident and secure
with my eating habits, my weight, and my continued commitment to my health and happiness. I started to make
new goals. My journal was about new things I wanted to
accomplish.

—Tricia

Many Reverse Dieters find they have the time and energy to shift their focus away from weight issues to new goals or hobbies in their lives. After the bridge phase and once in the Reverse Diet for Life Maintenance Phase, many Reverse Dieters are over their fear of reintroducing foods into their diets that might not be on the Reverse Diet Food List. They are confident as they look toward the rest of their lives and plan to maintain their results for the long run. Keeping your Reverse lifestyle in perspective and maintaining it for an extended amount of time is what the third phase of the plan is about. At this point, you know you'll be able to maintain the results you've seen because your healthy habits have become second nature. You now own your Reverse Diet skills.

The New Reverse You

When you compare the person who began the Reverse Diet with the person you are now, you'll see the distinct change not only in your weight but also in your approach to health and the way you perceive food. No longer is food an object to be lusted after or obsessed with—something that makes you feel guilty or inadequate. Food is no longer a scary subject for you in this phase. While you still may be apprehensive, confidence, a good self-image, and a different way of eating have helped you enrich the quality of your life and have reframed your outlook. Food will help you fuel the life you want, look the way you want, enjoy good health, and have energy rather than serving as a detrimental focus that contributes to weight cycling, and as a distraction from larger issues going on.

When you started phase one, you may have been in a very different state, mentally and emotionally:

- Before, you might have habitually eaten processed, high-fat, high-sugar, or salty foods. Now you automatically examine labels when at the store and try to prepare or seek out nutritious whole foods.

- Before, you might have been overwhelmed by all of the information and popular diets about what's healthy and what's not—when to avoid this and when to avoid that. Now you feel educated about what's healthy and what helps your body function better.

• Before, you might have regularly engaged in unhealthy cycles that included overeating, bingeing, and low self-esteem, guilt or shame, followed by trying to compensate with unhealthy or unrealistic dieting, skipping meals and repeating the cycle over and over. Now you rarely beat yourself up when you occasionally overeat and you have broken the yo-yo cycles that seemed to control your life before.

• Before, you might have allowed your emotions to determine when and how you overate. Now you notice those emotions and are aware that they do not have to have a negative effect on your food selections.

• Before, you thought many of your problems would be solved by reaching a goal weight or clothing size. Now you realize problems are easier to solve when paying mindful, careful attention to a healthy lifestyle, including better sleep, time management, good communication, and sound financial management.

• Before, you might have thought a perfect weight would make you happier. Now you realize that has more to do with your outlook, your actions, and your self-image.

• Before, you may have continued eating regardless of your body signals. Now you pay attention to hunger and fullness and can distinguish psychological cues to eat from physical cues to eat.

Here are some simple, specific changes that Tricia noticed in her lifestyle when she went into the third, maintenance, phase:

• Ordering takeout or at a restaurant, I automatically know what foods to choose and how they are prepared. I've learned that there are choices other than just pizza, subs, and fried dumplings on a takeout menu.

• When going to a function, I automatically call ahead to get the menu so I am prepared, or I bring my own food.

- I have no problem politely telling someone who might be serving unhealthy food when I am a guest somewhere that "I do not eat these kinds of food" or that I'm allergic to oil, chocolate, and so on, so that I may politely decline an overzealous host or hostess. I am prepared for any situation now. I don't allow a situation to control me; I control the situation.

- Now I know how to ride out a plateau or adjust my intake or activity to get past it.

- When I go shopping, I know my grocery store route and my favorite Reverse Diet foods so well that I do not even need a shopping list anymore. (**Note:** It takes a long time to get to this place; don't be discouraged if you still need to plan—it's important that you use planning to assist your new lifestyle as long as you need it.)

- I know how to stock my kitchen with the right foods to fix my favorite meals and favorite snacks.

- My menu and meal choices are creative—I can tweak any recipe and make it Reverse Diet Food List friendly.

- I automatically recognize portion sizes. Now I don't need to measure my meat, and there is no question what a small, medium, or large potato looks like or what a proper serving of pasta, pizza, or dessert is.

- A bakery is overwhelming for me now—everything smells and tastes way too sweet. I don't enjoy salty or sugary, processed foods; they are too rich for my everyday consumption. I eat them rarely on special occasions.

- My metabolism is in high gear. I can burn food more efficiently than when I had an unhealthy lifestyle.

- My immune system is better—I rarely get sick.

- I have more energy to participate in my life more fully.

- As I have freed up space from obsessing or thinking about food (what I was going to eat, what I had eaten, etc.), I have gained more mental energy to put into my career, family, and life.

REVERSE DIET EXERCISE

Take Stock of Your Changes

Take a moment with your journal. Look at the original goal you had when you first began the Reverse Diet. What have you learned since? How much more have you gotten besides just losing pounds?

Take a moment to write your own before-and-after changes.

A Reverse Relationship with Weight Gain

At this point, many Reverse Dieters have seen their bodies go from an unhealthy state to a healthy one. One Reverse Dieter, Teresa, said about the third phase,

It was how marathoners must feel when they finish a race—I went through so much. Not only was my body different, but I was different. I had overcome so many of the personal obstacles that had made me overweight. I went from an original weight of 268 to 172. I'm 5'8½". Some might think I'm still 'big,' but I feel great about myself. It took losing all that weight to realize that it's not about food or weight—success is about my happiness. I had been a little smaller during the bridge phase, about 155, but this is a more realistic weight for me. I even get more compliments now than I did then, and I think that's because I feel so wonderful about myself. My body image has changed for the better.

Tricia had a similar experience. She says,

One summer I got to 112, way too thin. Then I got my weight up to 138 the next summer. 112 was much too small for my 5'8" frame so I was told to gain some weight by my doctor. I worried. With a free pass to eat what I wanted, would I fall into my old bad eating habits? I was cautious and I ate higher-calorie foods that were still healthy, and I made sure I gained the weight back slowly. Eventually I went a little over my goal weight and then I went back on the plan to get it off. The most important discovery for me was this: I was not scared of gaining because I knew I could get it back off. My weight loss was not a fluke—the Reverse Diet really worked.

Knowing you can lose weight and that you can *maintain* a healthy weight is the real goal of the Reverse Diet for Life phase. Finding your balance, your center, a range of weight that's just right, can be tough—too much or too little can make you feel off kilter. Like a child riding a bike without training wheels for the first time or a ballerina learning how to stand on one toe, it is about experimenting and correcting until you find your center weight that helps you keep your balance.

When Reverse Dieters feel confident they can gain 5 pounds but it doesn't lead to the same life they had before, they are closer to having a balanced weight and a balanced lifestyle. The mind-set should be that if you gain 5 pounds, you need to take action and get back to the basics of healthy eating. You adjust, you do not panic and overeat.

Continuing the Reverse Diet Way of Life

Just because you have accomplished what you set out to do doesn't mean you can stop what you've learned on the Reverse Diet. Tricia, along with many Reverse Dieters, continues to journal every day. This keeps her mindful about her mental state and her outlook, how she approaches eating, and what goals she sets for herself. It also helps her keep tuned in to her body. By checking in with herself on a daily basis, she always remains in touch with how she responds to hunger, what types of habits are developing, and when her old habits reoccur.

There are other reasons to use your journal, too. Tricia says, "A lot of times, what I write is not so much about every food I eat. Sometimes it can be more about my daily goals and the activities I want to accomplish for that day. I do not use it as I would a daily planner, but it keeps me committed to what I said I was going to do, and at the end of the day I make my check marks on all that I followed through on."

Don't write only when you've had a bad eating day. It's helpful to check in regularly so you can keep in touch with yourself and what's really going on, and so you can provide yourself with the information to look back and see what patterns emerge.

Many Reverse Dieters seek motivation to continue their new lifestyles through the Reverse Diet Web site (reversedietsolution .com), and communicate with others on the diet at all stages.

Reverse Your Focus: The Rest of the Pie

One of the most important parts of success on the Reverse Diet is figuring out what besides weight loss can and will improve in your life. Let's revisit a concept from the beginning of the book. Keep the other areas of your life in mind as well—they can be family, social, cultural, career, spiritual, physical, personal development, aesthetic, intellectual, financial, and other goals. Now that weight loss and achieving a positive self-image are no longer your main goals, what can you put your energy toward? What other parts of life need attention and focus? You may decide, for instance, that culture takes a back seat when your kids are young, or to put your career on hold for the moment. Any decision is fine as long as it is a thoughtful one rather than just because you're in such disarray you can't think.

Tricia experienced this when she made it to the Reverse Diet for Life phase. She found herself more comfortable in all sorts of relationships, from romantic to social. "My relationships with others changed. I began a new relationship with my husband—I felt happier in our marriage, more intimate." With her daughters, instead of feeling helpless and overwhelmed, she says, "My relationship with my kids changed. I got involved in a ton of school programs. I was more conscious of their eating, and began teaching them to eat like I eat—healthfully. As a family, we went on vacation more. I was ready to be active, go swimming. I wasn't afraid of a bathing suit and was looking forward to enjoying an active, adventurous vacation with my family." Socially, she was brave in new adventures she had been afraid of before. "I found new friends and I was getting out more. I was more confident and outgoing. It changed my whole social life! Being 130 instead of almost 300 pounds can really change the way you see yourself through others' eyes."

The way Tricia dressed changed, too. "My choice in clothing is different—I love to dress up, wear suits, and a bikini! I had direction, was motivated and motivating, more confident. Ultimately my new wardrobe symbolized my new feeling that I wasn't afraid to really *live* life. These days, I try to experience all I can."

She also found herself putting more energy into what she wanted to do with her life. Before she lost weight, she was reluctant to break out of her old routine because she had low energy—now she had more energy, and her newfound confidence helped her address her desire for a career change. "My career changed from the nursing industry to the weight-loss and motivating industry. I wanted to help others achieve the same goals I had. It felt good to spread the positive experience I had, how I had learned to reverse my life—to virtually turn my self-esteem upside down, for the better."

Every Reverse Diet success story is different. One Reverse Dieter, Thomas, is an attorney who built a business through years of high pressure and long hours of hard work. The long hours at the desk and stress drove him to overeat, and he was overweight for many years. After losing weight and adopting a healthier, balanced diet, he began focusing on other things besides work. Although he could not completely abandon his job at the firm since he depended on it financially, he tried to take on more cases pro bono and work on houses for Habitat for Humanity a few times a month. This helped him broaden his scope from just work and diet to other things that boosted his confidence, enriched his life, and expanded his world view.

Spiritually, Tricia has found herself more thankful than ever before. "Instead of saying 'Why me? What have I done to deserve this unhappiness?' I say, 'I am thankful for everything I have.'"

REVERSE DIET EXERCISE

Focus on Your Goals Anew

What are your Reverse for Life goals? Grab your journal and list what you'd like to do now that you've reached a place with your body that empowers you rather than making you feel powerless.

Ask yourself what other parts of your life you want to focus on now that you have a more positive self-image and don't have to focus full time on weight loss or food. Maybe you have a relationship in your family you would like to nurture more? Perhaps you have a degree or a course you'd like to pursue for fun or profit? Maybe you have wanted to pursue a different career path and have never felt you had the time or were worthy? Now that you've conquered the weight challenge, there is no better time than the present!

Find a New Identity

Often when Reverse Dieters get to this phase, they find a new identity they may not have had at the beginning of the first phase. This can mean all sorts of things. With Tammy, when she weighed 230 pounds, her identity had been shrouded in shame and in her inability to stop overeating. She had a tough time figuring out what else she wanted from life because she was so focused on trying not to overeat and then feeling terrible when she would overeat. She didn't wear clothes that made her feel good, she wasn't very social, and she rented movies or watched TV in her free time instead of seeing people.

After she finished the Reverse Diet plan, her weight had gone down to 160. With a 5'8" frame, she felt terrific about herself. After learning how to flip-flop her meals, she found this was a comfortable, appropriate weight for herself—one where she could eat healthy and satisfying meals. The fact that she could control her eating enabled her to uncover a boisterous, outgoing woman who wanted to explore things she had never done before. She was braver about entertaining and meeting new friends, and she felt great in her clothes. A whole new world opened up to her now that she wasn't consumed with her eating habits or her poor body image. She began to travel any chance she got, and she set a goal for herself—to visit every state in the country. She's now on her thirtieth state and she's having a great time.

As you find balance in your life and weight cycling, you may also find others who are inspired by your success. As Tricia discovered, her new body and lifestyle motivated her daughter to take control of her weight, too. She says:

My oldest daughter, Brittni, has always fluctuated with her weight and she had developed emotional eating habits. At times she would even go so far as to hide food under her bed and then ask for seconds. I was in a predicament because I had already lost a lot of weight on the Reverse Diet. I knew that she was overeating but I didn't want to deny my child if she was hungry.

I knew that Brittni was using food to comfort herself. By the time I realized what was really happening, she was starting to gain weight. It was especially hard for her because I was doing so well and spreading news about the Reverse Diet while she still felt overweight.

While I could help her with her eating at home, I could not when she was away at grandma's house or at school. Finally Brittni became boy crazy and she came to me and asked, 'Mum, can you help me lose weight?' I was so proud of her and realized she had just had her Reverse Moment. We sat down together and came up with a game plan. While she ate a big breakfast at home that I made, she needed to really be educated on food choices when she was at school and when she visited friends and family for dinner. We worked on cutting out extra snacks, chips, and candy. She stopped drinking so many sodas and artificial fruit drinks. She learned about portion control and how to recognize food cravings versus actual hunger.

Brittni started her new lifestyle change at 160 pounds at age thirteen at 5'5" and I am proud to say that through all of her hard work and determination, she is now down to a healthy 134 pounds and happy as a lark. We went shopping for bathing suits a few weeks ago and Brittni has a beautiful blue two-piece. I notice that she has more energy and watches less TV. Of course she has the occasional pizza or candy with her friends. But now, instead of eating a whole pizza or bag of chips at once, she'll stop eating when she's full. I am so proud of my daughter and she is proud of herself!

Celebration Time!

As you work toward your life goals, be sure to reward yourself. You've learned to reward yourself for short-term goals, but for those long-term goals discussed in chapter 5, figure out a way to reward yourself for achieving a balanced weight and a healthy lifestyle. You deserve it. Continue to take the focus off food-based rewards. Other rewards can include all sorts of things, from taking some much-needed quality time with your family to pursuing a dream!

Give Away Your Comfort Outfit

Do you have a comfort outfit that you used to wear when you felt self-conscious and didn't want to wear an outfit that would fit your body? Reverse Dieters often describe this outfit as black or of a very bland color and very loose fitting. Everyone has something they wear when they aren't feeling all that great about themselves and usually it's less than flattering. Now that you're in phase three, we encourage you to give it away to charity or toss that outfit if you haven't already done so! Make a ceremony out of it. Maybe give it away and then give yourself a little pat on the back by taking a trip to your favorite store, treating yourself to an afternoon with your friends, or even toasting yourself with a glass of your favorite wine. Do something that marks the occasion—out with the old and in with the new!

Get Yourself a New Wardrobe

One of the first things Tricia did was to buy a new wardrobe for her new physique. It's not about fashion, it's about the fact that you can wear clothes you may not have been able to wear before. Your confidence will soar when you pick up smaller clothes sizes, especially if you weren't able to shop at certain stores before. Just trying on clothes will be more fun than the old negative cycle that might have followed clothes shopping before you became a Reverse Dieter. Now you'll be able to leave a store feeling good instead of bad whether you buy anything or not.

If the thought of spending money is daunting, don't agonize about it or put your bank account in the red zone—buy an accessory or just one piece of inexpensive clothing that you love. You can do what Tricia did—she went shopping at Goodwill and got a bunch of fun clothes that she could wear without spending much at all.

Remaking your wardrobe for your new lifestyle should be fun as you explore colors and styles that are new to you. One Reverse Dieter, Melissa, said of her new wardrobe, "I bought pinks, yellows, and greens with patterns I never would have worn before. I used to wear loose clothes and baggy, elastic pants in brown, beige, and black. Then I realized that green really accentuates my green eyes. Now I wear it all the time."

If you don't want to remake your wardrobe, remake something else! Redecorate a room in your house or celebrate your change in life with an adventure. One Reverse Dieter, Rob, bought a bike and started taking bike rides after work. Before, he felt too heavy to be comfortable on a bike. Now he says, "I never thought of myself as athletic or physically able to do anything active. Now I love to ride my bike after work or on the weekends. It takes the place of eating big dinners."

Throw a Big Loser Party

Tricia had a big party after she lost her weight and she encourages all Reverse Dieters to do the same. By letting themselves celebrate their accomplishments, many dieters feel they've reached a benchmark. Tricia explains:

> My anniversary date is March 17, which also happens to be St. Patrick's Day, so each year I celebrate two events on that date. My first was 2001, and a ton of us from work had a party. They all knew this was a huge milestone for me, too, my first anniversary. It was incredible; I made my own shirt out of a gold material and bought a pair of shiny green slacks. The outfit was so cute and I felt great. I make sure that I keep a picture from my party every year, even if it's just a quiet little celebration. It's a constant reminder of my achievement.

At your Big Loser party, there can be all kinds of celebrations and it doesn't have to revolve around food and alcohol. It can have more to do with learning to have fun at parties in different ways from before. For example, one Reverse Dieter, Harriet, got interested in knitting while on the plan. She would knit every chance she got, especially when she felt like eating something she shouldn't. Harriet loves to have knitting parties. There is no alcohol or unhealthy food; the party is just focused toward being with friends and having fun.

Tricia found that making herself healthier helped her family get healthier, too. Now her husband can come to the Big Loser party, too. She says:

> My husband, Sean, and I were brought together over four and a half years ago. At the beginning of our relationship he was 6'2" and weighed 265 pounds. After losing all of my weight, I had a new Reverse Diet lifestyle. I was still respectful of his way of eating, though, and did not push my new lifestyle on him or lecture him, I just continued the Reverse Diet to maintain my new weight.

He would try to get me to eat whatever he was having for dinner and even went as far as to complain that I did not eat 'right' or 'normal,' or he'd lovingly tease me. Sometimes I ate poorly just to make him happy. He did not understand the concept of the Reverse Diet. It took a few years, but in the end I won. After he moved in with me and my daughters, he realized that my cupboards and refrigerator were his, too. He began to eat the foods on the Reverse Diet.

Although he does not follow the plan to a T and I really do not know if he ever will, after being in the house he is now down to 212 pounds and he has joined the gym. He has also learned how to read food labels, about the unhealthy effects of consuming too much sodium, and not to plan a large dinner at seven o'clock with friends and family.

Every once in a while, when I go out of town, my family still has a burger or chips. They treat themselves to the occasional flub. Even so, overall they have adapted to the new lifestyle very well. Sean has even learned how to go shopping for our Reverse Diet lifestyle—he knows what products are healthy and the ones that are not!

I've begun to coach my father, too, and I've shown him how to shop and plan meals. He has been following the concept for the past two months and has lost 25 pounds!

Just as the diet can be personalized, so can your Reverse Diet for Life. What do you want to do with your life that you didn't do before? It doesn't have to be about clothes, or weight, or exercise. It can be *anything* that makes you feel good. Your new way of life is about acknowledging all the emotions and reactions that accompany eating and your self-image and choosing to act or not to act on them. You are now on your way to gaining the skills you need for the life you want. You're on your way to a whole new world of possibilities. Congratulations!

9

Reverse Diet Recipes

In this chapter, you'll find some of Tricia's favorite recipes. They have been used by successful Reverse Dieters to achieve the results they want. Many of the recipes in this chapter use salt and sugar substitutes. Tricia's favorites are AlsoSalt and Splenda; yours may vary. Have fun when you cook, and make it a hobby! Cooking can be almost as fun as eating.

MAIN COURSES

Reverse Diet Cereal Mix

Serves 1

½ cup oatmeal, uncooked
½ cup shredded wheat, bite-size or biscuit-size with no sugar
4 to 6 ounces orange juice, no-sugar-added cranberry juice, or
    prune juice
1 banana or other fruit (optional)

In a bowl mix together the oatmeal and shredded wheat. After mixing, pour your choice of juice over the mixture. You may add a banana or your favorite fruit.

Reverse Diet Breakfast Wrap

Makes 2 servings

½ medium onion, chopped
1 cup peppers (red, yellow, and green), diced
1 tablespoon minced garlic
½ tomato, diced
1 teaspoon parsley
2 slices firm tofu, crumbled
2 tablespoons lemon juice
½ teaspoon black pepper
4 eggs
2 large lettuce or cabbage leaves
fat-free sour cream or your favorite dressing (optional)

In a medium saucepan mix all the ingredients except the eggs and lettuce or cabbage, cover with a lid, and cook over medium heat until the vegetables are soft. Then add the eggs, stirring frequently, and cook until the eggs are firm and thoroughly cooked. Place your choice of lettuce or cabbage leaves on a plate. Spoon half of the mixture onto each leaf. Starting at the top, fold the leaf up, then fold the right side, then the left, and roll it up until you have formed your wrap. Add fat-free sour cream or your favorite dressing on the side.

Garlic Breath Tip

After eating garlic, eat a fresh sprig of parsley. Its breath-neutralizing process has been known for centuries and was there before mints and toothpaste.

Reverse Diet Veggie Burger

Serves 2

⅔ cup tofu, crumbled
1   cup cooked lentils
½   cup cooked garbanzo beans
1   cup portabello mushrooms, roasted and minced
1   tablespoon minced garlic
1   cup crushed shredded wheat
½   medium onion, minced
2   eggs
extra-virgin olive oil

Heat the grill or broiler. Mix together all the ingredients except the oil in a large bowl and refrigerate for ½ hour. Form the mixture into patties and brush each with the oil. Grill or broil for 5 to 10 minutes until the patties are hot in the middle.

Reverse Diet Stuffed Green Peppers

Serves 4

1   pound lean ground turkey
1   medium onion, diced
½ cup diced celery
½ teaspoon white pepper
1   teaspoon thyme
1½ cups instant brown rice, cooked
4   large green peppers, tops sliced and seeds removed
2   medium tomatoes, puréed in a blender
2   tablespoons Parmesan cheese

Preheat the oven to 375 degrees. In a large skillet, brown the turkey until it is thoroughly cooked and no longer pink. Then add the onion, celery, white pepper, and thyme, simmering until the vegetables are tender. Add the rice to the turkey and vegetable mixture.

Stuff the peppers with the mixture and stand upright in a deep-dish baking pan with ¼ inch of water on the bottom. Pour the puréed tomatoes over each pepper and sprinkle with the Parmesan cheese. Cover with a lid or aluminum foil and bake for 30 to 40 minutes or until the peppers are soft.

Reverse Diet Stuffed Tuna Tofu Tomatoes

Serves 2

2   medium tomatoes
1   can chunk light tuna in water, drained
½ cup fat-free sour cream

1   chopped red onion
½   cup chopped celery
1   teaspoon black pepper
½   cubed extra-firm tofu

Slice off the tops of the tomatoes and scoop out the insides and place to the side. In a large bowl, combine the rest of the ingredients, mixing them until all are folded thoroughly. Spoon the mixture into the cored tomatoes and place on a bed of fresh greens, using the insides of the tomatoes as a garnish.

Reverse Diet Southern Shrimp Creole

Serves 4

1   medium onion, chopped
¾   cup chopped celery
½   cup green pepper
½   cup red sweet pepper
½   cup hot banana pepper
1   cup diced tomatoes
1   tablespoon parsley
½   teaspoon cayenne pepper
½   teaspoon black pepper
2   tablespoons minced garlic
½   cup cold water
2   teaspoons cornstarch
1   pound fresh or frozen shrimp, deveined and with tails removed
2   cups instant brown rice, cooked

REVERSE DIET SOUTHERN SHRIMP CREOLE (*CONTINUED*)

In a saucepan combine the onion, celery, all peppers, tomatoes, parsley, cayenne pepper, black pepper, and garlic. Cook over medium heat until the vegetables are soft. In a small bowl mix together the water and cornstarch, and then mix in the shrimp.

Combine the mixture with the vegetables and spices in the saucepan. Cook, simmering, until the sauce thickens and the shrimp are no longer translucent. Serve over the rice.

Reverse Diet Southern "Fried" Chicken

Serves 4

½   cup rolled oats
¼   cup crushed shredded wheat
½   cup mashed potato flakes
1   teaspoon garlic powder
½   teaspoon onion powder
¼   teaspoon black pepper
¼   teaspoon ground red pepper (optional)
1   tablespoon Parmesan cheese
2   eggs
4   tablespoons ultra-fat-free skim milk
4   boneless, skinless chicken breasts
nonstick cooking spray

Preheat the oven to 400 degrees. In a bowl, mix the oats, shredded wheat, potato flakes, garlic powder, onion powder, black pepper, red pepper, and Parmesan cheese. Transfer to a 2-quart plastic bag.

In another bowl, beat the eggs and milk together. Submerge the chicken breasts in the egg mixture, then add them to the breading bag, seal, and shake. It is important to do one breast at a time. Lay the chicken on a flat baking sheet that has been sprayed with the cooking spray. Bake for 35 minutes or until cooked through.

Reverse Diet Chicken Melt

Serves 1

½ lemon
1   5-ounce chicken breast
dash oregano and parsley
2   slices tomato
3   strips green pepper
4   sliced onion rings
1   low-fat Swiss cheese slice

Preheat the oven to 370 degrees. In a bowl, squeeze the lemon over the chicken, season with the oregano and parsley, and refrigerate for ½ hour. Remove the chicken and place in a 9 × 13-inch baking dish and fill the dish with ½ inch of water. On top of the chicken place the rest of the ingredients except the cheese. Cover and bake for 45 minutes. When the chicken is done add the cheese and broil for 20 to 30 seconds on the center rack until the cheese is melted.

Reverse Diet Sloppy Toms

Serves 6

1   pound ground turkey
1   medium onion, diced
1   medium green pepper, diced
1   cup puréed tomatoes, seeds removed
1   tablespoon dry mustard

2   teaspoons low-sodium Worcestershire sauce
¼   teaspoon cayenne pepper
6   low-sodium, low-calorie whole wheat hamburger
    buns
6   slices low-fat Swiss cheese

Brown the turkey, onion, and pepper in a medium skillet until the turkey is no longer pink, then drain. Add the tomatoes, mustard, Worcestershire, and cayenne pepper to the turkey, and simmer for 15 to 20 minutes.

Spoon Sloppy Toms onto the hamburger buns, and place one slice of Swiss cheese on each sandwich.

Reverse Diet Simply Salmon

Serves 1

1   6-ounce portion of salmon
2   tablespoons extra-virgin olive oil
1   teaspoon dill
¼   teaspoon oregano
1   teaspoon parsley
2   slices lemon

Preheat the oven to 350 degrees. Place the salmon in a baking dish. In a bowl, mix the oil, dill, oregano, and parsley. Brush the mixture over the salmon. Top the salmon with the lemon. Cover and bake for 20 to 25 minutes.

Reverse Diet Shrimp
a la Queen

Serves 6

¼ cup low-fat, low-sodium butter substitute
1   green pepper, diced
½ cup sliced mushrooms
½ cup minced onion
3   tablespoons whole wheat flour
2   tablespoons minced garlic
½ teaspoon black pepper
2   cups skim milk
2   cups cooked shrimp
1   cup shredded part-skim mozzarella cheese
3   cups brown rice, cooked

In a large saucepan at medium heat sauté the butter substitute, green pepper, mushrooms, and onion. Lower the heat, then stir in the flour, garlic, and black pepper, and gradually add the milk. Add the shrimp and stir constantly until the mixture thickens, then remove the mixture from the heat. Stir in the mozzarella cheese, and when melted, pour the mixture over ½ cup rice on each serving dish.

Reverse Diet Rice
Cake Pizza

Serves 2

1   tomato, puréed
¼ teaspoon oregano
1   teaspoon garlic

> dash black pepper
> 2 rice cakes
> ½ cup finely diced small onion
> 1 1-ounce slice tofu, diced
> 1 slice provolone cheese

Preheat the oven to 400 degrees. Mix the tomato, oregano, garlic, and black pepper and spread evenly on both rice cakes. On top of the mixture, add the onion, tofu, and one slice of cheese per pizza. Bake for 10 minutes.

Reverse Diet Piggyback Enchiladas

Serves 10

10 low-sodium whole wheat tortillas
1 pound lean ground pork loin
1 large onion, chopped
3 tablespoons minced jalapeño peppers (optional)
1 teaspoon cayenne pepper
½ teaspoon black pepper
1 teaspoon cilantro
1 green pepper, chopped
1 sweet pepper, chopped
2 tomatoes, chopped
½ cup part-skim mozzarella cheese, shredded
1 head of iceberg lettuce, shredded
8-ounce container fat-free sour cream

Preheat the oven to 350 degrees. Place the tortillas in aluminum foil and bake for 5 minutes or until the tortillas are just starting to brown. In a large skillet combine the ground pork loin, onion, jalapeño peppers, cayenne pepper, black pepper, cilantro, green pepper, and sweet pepper. Cook over medium heat until the meat is brown, then drain.

Spoon some of the pork mixture into the middle of each tortilla. Add 2 tablespoons of the tomatoes and the mozzarella cheese. Then roll up the tortillas and place them in a large deep-dish pan with a toothpick securing the seam. Bake them for 15 to 20 minutes.

When the tortillas are done, place the shredded lettuce on each dish and set a burrito on top. Add a dollop of sour cream and serve. (Optional: Lettuce is always a good substitute for a tortilla.)

Reverse Diet
Meat Loaf

Serves 6 to 8

2   pounds lean ground turkey
2   eggs
1   medium onion, chopped
1   medium green pepper, chopped
¾   cup shredded wheat, crushed
2   tablespoons Parmesan cheese
1   teaspoon oregano
1   tomato, diced
2   tablespoons minced garlic
½   cup no-salt-added ketchup

Preheat the oven to 350 degrees. Mix all the ingredients, except the ketchup, in a large bowl. Shape the mixture into a loaf with a large spoon. Place the loaf in a pan or casserole dish, baste with the ketchup, and add ¼ inch of water on the bottom of the pan. Cover and bake for 45 minutes to 1 hour, until cooked.

Reverse Diet Mac and Cheese Bake

Serves 6

¼ cup low-fat, low-sodium butter substitute
1   large onion, diced
⅛ cup whole wheat flour
3   cups skim milk
½ box elbow macaroni, cooked
1½ cups part-skim mozzarella, shredded
yellow food coloring (optional)
1   large tomato, diced
2   tablespoons Parmesan cheese

Melt the butter substitute in a 4-quart saucepan over medium heat and add the onion until carmelized (slightly browned), then stir in the flour and cook for 2 to 3 minutes. Add the milk and stir while bringing the mixture to a simmer. Combine the pasta, cover, and continue to simmer gently for 4 to 5 minutes, stirring occasionally until the mixture thickens. Remove the mixture from the heat and add the cheese, stirring until the cheese is melted. Add a few drops of the food coloring for a more traditional look. Pour the mixture into a 1½-quart casserole dish. Add the tomato and bake at 350 degrees, uncovered, for 30 minutes. Garnish with the Parmesan cheese.

Reverse Diet Jambalaya

Serves 2

¾ cup chopped onion
½ cup chopped celery
¼ cup chopped red sweet pepper
¼ cup green pepper

4   tablespoons minced garlic
2   tomatoes, diced
2   tablespoons low-fat, low-sodium butter substitute
2   cups water
¾   cup instant long grain brown rice, uncooked
¼   teaspoon cayenne pepper
¼   cup chopped hot banana pepper (optional)
1   8-ounce chicken breast, diced small
1   pound fresh or frozen (thawed) peeled shrimp

In a large saucepan add all the ingredients, except the chicken and shrimp, and bring to a boil; cover and simmer for 20 minutes. Add the chicken and shrimp, cover, and simmer for 20 more minutes or until the chicken is cooked through.

Reverse Diet Italian Chicken

Serves 1

1   4-6-ounce chicken breast

Italian Sauce

½   teaspoon oregano
1   tablespoon extra-virgin olive oil
½   teaspoon Parmesan cheese
½   teaspoon basil
1   teaspoon minced garlic

Heat a grill. Mix all the ingredients for the Italian sauce in a bowl. Make three tiny cuts on the top of the chicken breast and cover it with the sauce. Grill the chicken until it is no longer pink in the middle.

Reverse Diet Grumpy Grouper

Serves 4

1   pound fresh or frozen (thawed) grouper fish
¼   cup orange juice
½   teaspoon coarse black pepper
2   tablespoons finely chopped scallions
1   teaspoon minced chili pepper
¼   teaspoon dry mustard
1   teaspoon dill
2   tablespoons lemon juice
1   cup fat-free sour cream

Preheat the oven on broil. Dry the grouper with paper towels. Place the fish in a baking dish with the orange juice and broil for 8 to 10 minutes. While the fish is cooking, mix all the other ingredients together in a large bowl. When the fish is done and flaky, pour the mixture over the grouper and place it under the broiler for 2 to 5 minutes.

Reverse Diet Fettuccine and Asparagus

Serves 2

½   box (8 ounces) whole wheat fettuccine noodles
2   tablespoons low-fat, low-sodium butter substitute, divided
1   tablespoon minced garlic

1 cup fresh or frozen asparagus, whole
1 tablespoon lemon juice
8 tablespoons Parmesan cheese
½ teaspoon coarse black pepper
1 teaspoon parsley

Fill a large pot ¾ full of water and bring to a boil over high heat. When the water has reached a full boil, add the noodles, cook until softened, and drain.

In a small pan melt 1 tablespoon of the butter substitute over medium heat. Add the garlic and asparagus and cook until the asparagus is slightly soft. Add the lemon juice, Parmesan cheese, black pepper, and parsley. Stir in the remaining butter substitute and cook another minute.

Place the noodles on a plate, then pour the sauce mixture over the noodles and top with the asparagus mix.

Reverse Diet Eggplant Lasagna

Serves 6

Sauce

6 medium tomatoes, peeled and diced
2 teaspoons minced garlic
1 teaspoon oregano
1 teaspoon parsley
¼ teaspoon chili pepper powder (optional)
½ teaspoon black pepper

REVERSE DIET EGGPLANT LASAGNA (*CONTINUED*)

Lasagna

- 2   whole eggplants, peeled and sliced thin
- 1   medium onion, diced
- 1   green pepper, diced
- 4   tablespoons Parmesan cheese
- ¾   cup low-fat ricotta cheese
- 1   8-ounce container fat-free sour cream
- 4   ounces of tofu
- 8   ounces shredded part-skim mozzarella

Place the peeled tomatoes in a medium saucepan and cook on medium heat until they are soft. Let the tomatoes cool and process them in a blender until they are liquefied. Pour the tomatoes into a mixing bowl, add the spices, and set aside.

Preheat the oven to 375 degrees. In a large saucepan parboil the eggplant slices for 10 minutes until they are soft, then drain and set aside. In a skillet, add the onion and green pepper and sauté until the vegetables are tender. In a bowl, combine the Parmesan cheese, ricotta, sour cream, and tofu.

In a 9 × 13-inch baking dish layer the ingredients using a third of the sauce, eggplant, and cheese mix for each layer. Add the mozzarella to the top of the lasagna, then cover and bake for 30 to 45 minutes.

Reverse Diet Egg Bake

Serves 8 to 10

- 1   cup fresh chopped broccoli
- 1   medium onion, chopped
- 1   green pepper, chopped

1   sweet red pepper, chopped
18 eggs
¾   cup skim milk
2   tablespoons minced garlic
1   teaspoon black pepper
½   cup part-skim mozzarella cheese

Preheat the oven to 450 degrees. In a saucepan over medium heat, sauté the broccoli, onion, and green and red peppers, until the peppers are soft.

Place the eggs and milk in a large bowl and whip until the eggs are smooth.

In a 9 × 13-inch greased glass baking dish, spoon in the vegetable mixture. Pour in the egg batter, and add the garlic and black pepper. Bake for 25 to 30 minutes until the top jiggles in the middle. Take a spatula and draw a line lengthwise across the middle until you see the egg batter seeping to the top. Spread the mozzarella cheese over the top and bake for an additional 5 to 10 minutes or until the middle is solid.

Reverse Diet Clucky Chicken Pot Pie

Serves 6

Pot Pie Center

4   cups water
2   medium potatoes, cubed
½   cup chopped carrots
½   cup chopped celery
2   boneless, skinless chicken breasts

REVERSE DIET CLUCKY CHICKEN POT PIE (*CONTINUED*)

- ¼ cup frozen corn
- ¼ cup frozen peas
- ¼ cup sliced mushrooms
- 1 tablespoon minced garlic
- ¼ cup nonfat yogurt
- ¼ cup skim milk
- 2 tablespoons whole wheat flour

Pot Pie Crusty Top

- 1 cup whole wheat flour
- 1 teaspoon baking powder
- 2 tablespoons low-fat, low-sodium butter substitute
- ½ cup skim milk

Preheat the oven to 350 degrees.

In a large saucepan, bring the water to a boil and add the potatoes, carrots, and celery, and simmer until the potatoes are soft. Add the chicken and cover and simmer for 20 to 30 minutes. Remove the chicken from the pot, drain, cool, and cut into cubes. Remove from the heat and add the rest of the vegetables and garlic, and set aside.

In a small pan over low heat, mix the yogurt and milk, slowly adding the whole wheat flour, stirring constantly until the mixture thickens. Remove from the heat and add the mixture to the vegetables and chicken. Pour the mixture into bowllike baking pans (you can use soup bowls that are oven safe).

To make the pie crust, in a medium bowl mix the whole wheat flour, baking powder, and butter substitute until smooth, then add the milk. Spoon the crust mixture into scoops on top of the pie center and spread evenly, making sure not to allow the crusty top to touch the sides. Bake for 45 minutes to 1 hour.

Reverse Diet Chili

Serves 4

1½ pounds ground turkey
4   tomatoes, diced into small pieces
2½ cups frozen red kidney beans
1   large green pepper, diced
1   large yellow pepper, diced
1   large onion, diced
3   tablespoons minced garlic
1   teaspoon black pepper
1   tablespoon lemon juice
1   teaspoon hot red pepper seeds (optional)

Brown the turkey in a skillet until it is no longer pink. Drain and set aside. In a large saucepan mix together all the ingredients except the turkey and simmer on medium heat until the vegetables are tender. Combine with the turkey and serve hot.

Reverse Diet Chicken and Tofu Stir Fry

Serves 1

2   tablespoons extra-virgin olive oil
1   boneless, skinless chicken breast
2   inches firm tofu, cut into small pieces
½   cup French-style green beans

½ small onion, sliced thin
½ tomato, cubed small
½ green pepper, diced small
handful of bean sprouts
2 teaspoons minced garlic
¼ teaspoon red pepper

Heat a medium skillet and add the olive oil, but don't let the oil smoke. Slice the chicken into cubes and brown in the skillet on medium heat until the chicken is no longer pink. Add the rest of the ingredients to the browned chicken and sauté until the vegetables are soft.

Reverse Diet Brown Rice and Tuna Casserole

Serves 4

2 cups brown rice, cooked
½ cup diced mushrooms
2 slices tofu, crumbled
½ cup frozen peas
1 6-ounce canned tuna, low-sodium, water-packed
8 ounces fat-free sour cream
¼ cup skim milk
2 tablespoons Parmesan cheese
⅔ cup crushed shredded wheat

Preheat the oven to 350 degrees. Mix all the ingredients except the shredded wheat together in a medium bowl and place in a casserole dish. Top with the shredded wheat. Cover and bake for 25 to 30 minutes. Remove the cover and bake for 15 minutes more.

Reverse Diet Artichoke Heart Casserole Medley

Serves 2

2   chicken breasts, diced
2   tablespoons olive oil
10 ounces fresh artichoke hearts, diced
1   cup sliced mushrooms
½   cup chopped red pepper
½   cup chopped yellow pepper
1   onion, diced
1   tomato, diced
½   teaspoon chili powder (optional)
2   teaspoons Parmesan cheese
1   teaspoon oregano
½   cup shredded wheat crumbs
3   eggs
½   cup fat-free sour cream
½   cup shredded provolone cheese
1   2-quart self-lock plastic bag

Preheat the oven to 350 degrees. Grill the chicken in a skillet with the olive oil on medium heat until it is no longer pink. In a separate skillet sauté the artichoke hearts, mushrooms, peppers, onion, tomato, chili powder, Parmesan cheese, and oregano. Cook on medium heat until the vegetables are soft. Add the chicken.

In a bowl mix the wheat crumbs, eggs, sour cream, and provolone cheese. Place the mixture in plastic bag and use a rolling pin to flatten it. Place the mixture in the casserole dish with the chicken, vegetables, and spices, and bake for 30 minutes.

Reverse Diet Scallops with Linguini in Tomato and Basil Sauce

Serves 4

1   pound whole wheat linguini
1   pound scallops
1   tablespoons extra-virgin olive oil
1   teaspoon of minced garlic
¼   cup white wine
2   tomatoes, diced
½   red sweet pepper, diced
½   green pepper, diced
½   yellow pepper, diced
½   teaspoon white pepper
1   tablespoon basil
½   teaspoon oregano

Cook the noodles according to the package directions, until soft. In a separate saucepan, sauté the scallops in the oil and garlic for about 2 minutes. Add the wine and sauté another 2 minutes. In another large skillet add all the vegetables and seasonings and sauté until the vegetables are tender. Pour the vegetable mixture over the pasta and add the scallops on top.

Reverse Diet Stuffed Zucchini

Serves 4

1 large zucchini
1 pound lean ground turkey
1 medium onion, diced
¼ cup shredded carrots
¼ cup diced mushrooms
½ cup red sweet peppers, diced
½ cup green bell pepper, diced
½ cup diced zucchini
2 tablespoons minced garlic
¼ teaspoon cayenne pepper
½ teaspoon black pepper
½ cup fat-free sour cream
2 puréed tomatoes
Parmesan cheese
½ cup shredded part-skim mozzarella

Preheat the oven to 400 degrees. Remove a ½-inch slice from the top of the zucchini lengthwise, scoop out the filling, and set aside. In a skillet, brown the turkey on medium heat until it is no longer pink. When the turkey is cooked, add all the vegetables and spices, except the tomatoes. After the meat and vegetables are mixed together, add the fat-free sour cream. Stuff the mixture into the zucchini and pour the tomatoes over the stuffed zucchini. Place in a deep-dish casserole pan or aluminum turkey pan with ¼ cup of water. Sprinkle the Parmesan cheese on top, then cover and bake for 25 minutes or until the zucchini is tender, then add the mozzarella cheese and bake 5 minutes more.

SIDE DISHES

Reverse Diet Twice-Stuffed Potatoes

Serves 4

4   medium potatoes
½ cup fat-free sour cream
1   tablespoon minced garlic
½ medium onion, minced
2   tablespoons skim milk
2   teaspoons Parmesan cheese
4   slices low-fat Swiss cheese

Preheat the oven to 425 degrees. Cook the potatoes in the microwave for 4 to 8 minutes or until a fork goes in easily. Let them stand for 10 to 15 minutes, then cut the tops off lengthwise and discard.

Scoop out the middles of the potatoes, place them in a bowl, and set aside. In another bowl, mix all the other ingredients except the Swiss cheese, and beat with electric beaters 3 to 5 minutes. Add the mix to the potato insides with a spoon, put the mixture back into the potato skins, and bake them for 20 to 25 minutes.

When the potatoes are done, place 1 slice of Swiss cheese on each potato and bake for 2 more minutes until the cheese is melted.

Reverse Diet Sweet Potatoes

Serves 4

4   large sweet potatoes, cut into small pieces
2   teaspoons cinnamon
¼   cup low-fat, low-sodium butter substitute
¼   teaspoon ginger

Preheat the oven to 400 degrees. Place the sweet potatoes in a casserole dish, adding the cinnamon, butter, and ginger on the top. Cover and bake for 1 hour or until the potatoes are soft.

Reverse Diet Stuffed Mushrooms with Crabmeat

Serves 8 to 10

1   6-ounce low-sodium can crabmeat or ½ pound of fresh, cooked crabmeat
2   teaspoons lemon juice
¼   cup nonfat yogurt
½   cup minced onions
1   teaspoon minced garlic
½   teaspoon thyme
24 medium mushrooms with stems removed

Preheat the oven to 400 degrees. Mix together all the ingredients except the mushrooms in a large bowl. Fill the mushroom caps with the mixture. Arrange the mushrooms on a baking sheet or baking dish and cover with aluminum foil. Bake for 12 to 15 minutes, remove the foil, and bake 5 more minutes until the mushrooms are golden brown.

Reverse Diet Stuffed Celery

Serves 2 to 4

1 to 2 8-ounce containers low-fat cottage cheese
½　pound crushed walnuts
1　teaspoon garlic powder
1　teaspoon onion powder
1　stalk celery, cut into 2-inch sections

Mix together the cream cheese, walnuts, garlic powder, and onion powder, and fill the celery sections with the mixture. Arrange on a dish or platter and serve.

Reverse Diet Cucumber Delights

Serves 4 to 6

4　cucumbers
1　16-ounce package of mushrooms, finely chopped
2　tablespoons olive oil
2　teaspoons lemon juice
1　tablespoon dill
1　teaspoon onion powder
1　teaspoon paprika for garnish

Peel the cucumbers and remove each end. Cut the cucumbers into 1-inch sections and scoop out the centers with a spoon. Set the cucumber insides aside.

In a saucepan, mix together all the other ingredients except the paprika, simmering over medium heat for 3 to 5 minutes. Drain the excess water and place the mixture in a bowl, cover, and chill. Before serving, fill the cucumber slices with the stuffing and top with the removed centers. Sprinkle with the paprika and serve.

Reverse Diet Salmon Roly-Polies

Serves 12

2   8-ounce packages fat-free cream cheese
6   tablespoons fat-free sour cream
1   teaspoon garlic powder
1   teaspoon onion powder
1   pound (12 slices) smoked, low-sodium salmon, thinly sliced
12 long-stemmed green onions, thinly sliced

In a large bowl mix together the cream cheese, sour cream, garlic powder, and onion powder, and set aside. Then lay each salmon slice out individually and spread the mixture evenly over each slice.

Add onions to each salmon slice and roll the slice up. Place on a serving platter and enjoy.

Reverse Diet Grilled Fruit Kabob with Cinnamon Sauce

Serves 4

Kabobs

4   apples, cubed
½   pineapple, cubed
4   pears, cubed
2   peaches, sectioned
2   oranges, peeled and sectioned
1   cup grapes
8   strawberries
8   wooden or metal skewers

REVERSE DIET GRILLED FRUIT KABOB WITH CINNAMON SAUCE
(*CONTINUED*)

Cinnamon Sauce

¾ cup lemon juice
¼ cup light brown sugar
1½ teaspoons cinnamon
1 teaspoon nutmeg
1 tablespoon vanilla extract

Preheat the grill or broiler to medium heat. Place pieces of the apples, pineapple, pears, peaches, oranges, grapes, and strawberries on skewers. If using the broiler, place the kabobs on a cookie sheet and set on the center rack.

Mix all the sauce ingredients together in a small bowl. Using a barbecue brush, lightly swab each fruit kabob until all are covered. Cook the kabobs for 5 to 7 minutes, turning often.

Reverse Diet Fried Zucchini

Serves 4

3 eggs
½ cup skim milk
4 tablespoons extra-virgin olive oil
1 large zucchini, sliced thin

Breading

1 cup crushed shredded wheat
1 teaspoon oregano
1 teaspoon parsley
1 teaspoon cilantro
1 teaspoon thyme

½ teaspoon rosemary
2 tablespoons Parmesan cheese
1 teaspoon black pepper

In a medium bowl mix together the eggs and milk to form a batter. In another bowl mix together all the breading ingredients.

Preheat the oil in a frying pan on medium heat. Dip the zucchini slices in the batter and then the breading, and place in the frying pan on medium-high heat, turning frequently until brown on both sides. Serve with your favorite Reverse Diet dip or dressing on the side.

Reverse Diet Scalloped Potatoes

Serves 4

4 potatoes, sliced thin
4 slices firm tofu
½ cup fat-free sour cream
¾ cup skim milk
4 tablespoons Parmesan cheese
2 teaspoons garlic
¼ cup minced onion
2 tablespoons parsley

Preheat the oven to 400 degrees. In a 9 × 13-inch baking dish spread the potatoes evenly. In a separate bowl add the tofu, sour cream, skim milk, Parmesan cheese, garlic, and onion, and mix with beaters on medium speed until the mixture is smooth and creamy. Pour the mixture over the potatoes in the baking dish and mix together. Sprinkle with the parsley, cover, and bake for 45 to 60 minutes or until the potatoes are tender.

Reverse Diet Coleslaw

Serves 2

1   8-ounce bag preshredded cabbage and carrot mix
1   medium onion, diced small
2   ounces fat-free sour cream
3   tablespoons apple cider vinegar
1   teaspoon minced garlic
¼   teaspoon vanilla
dash of ginger
½   teaspoon celery seed
½   teaspoon black pepper
¼   teaspoon crushed red pepper
1   tablespoon salt substitute
1   teaspoon sugar substitute

Place the cabbage and carrot mix and onion in a bowl and set aside. In a medium bowl mix the sour cream, vinegar, garlic, vanilla, ginger, celery seed, black pepper, red pepper, salt substitute, and sugar substitute. Add the cabbage mix. Chill for one hour in the refrigerator, then serve.

Reverse Diet Broccoli, Cauliflower, and Cheese

Serves 4

2   cups fresh or frozen broccoli, cut into small pieces
2   cups fresh or frozen cauliflower, cut into small pieces
1   cup nonfat yogurt
¼   cup skim milk
4   tablespoons Parmesan cheese
6   slices provolone cheese
1   teaspoon onion powder
2   tablespoons salt substitute

Preheat the oven to 350 degrees. In a casserole dish, mix together all the ingredients. Cover and bake for 35 minutes.

Reverse Diet South of the Border Fiesta on Corn Bread

Serves 6

Corn bread

1 cup whole wheat all-purpose flour
1 cup yellow cornmeal
1 teaspoon onion powder
1 teaspoon garlic powder
1 tablespoon baking powder
¼ cup low-fat, low-sodium butter substitute
1 cup skim milk
1 egg
nonstick cooking spray

Refried beans

½ cup extra-virgin olive oil
2 cups frozen pinto beans, thawed
2 tablespoons chili powder
1 tablespoon ground cumin
1 teaspoon onion powder
1 teaspoon garlic powder
1 teaspoon salt substitute
⅛ teaspoon pepper

Fiesta mix

1 cup diced tomatoes
½ cup frozen corn, slightly cooked and drained
1 large onion, finely chopped
2 chili peppers, finely chopped
1 large green pepper, diced
1 tablespoon minced garlic
½ cup shredded part-skim mozzarella cheese
fat-free sour cream

Preheat the oven to 400 degrees. In a medium bowl mix together the flour, cornmeal, onion powder, garlic powder, and baking powder. Place the butter substitute in a small container and melt in the microwave for about 30 to 40 seconds, then add it to a separate bowl with the milk and egg. Beat the mixture together until well combined, then add it to the flour mixture and stir until a smooth batter forms. Coat the inside of a 9 × 13-inch baking dish with the nonstick cooking spray and pour the batter into the dish. Bake for 15 to 20 minutes until the top is golden brown. Stick a toothpick in the center; when there is no batter sticking to the toothpick, the bread is done. Remove the corn bread and let it cool on a baking rack.

Heat the oil in a large skillet over medium heat and add the pinto beans, stirring occasionally for about 5 minutes. Smash the beans and stir in the chili powder, cumin, onion powder, garlic powder, salt substitute, and pepper, mixing together until a paste forms. Spread the refried bean mixture over the cooled corn bread.

In a large bowl combine all the fiesta mix ingredients. Spread the mixture over the top of the refried beans and bake for 25 minutes. Add a dollop of fat-free sour cream on top of each serving.

SALADS

Reverse Diet Pasta Salad

Serves 8

4   cups whole wheat rotini pasta
½   medium cucumber, chopped
½   medium zucchini, chopped

1 large tomato, diced, seeds removed
1 medium green pepper, diced
1 medium sweet red pepper, diced
½ medium onion, diced
2 ounces tofu, crumbled
¼ cup shredded part-skim mozzarella cheese

Dressing

¼ cup water
¼ cup vinegar
4 tablespoons extra-virgin olive oil
1 tablespoon basil
½ teaspoon oregano
½ teaspoon black pepper

Cook the noodles according to the package directions. Drain the pasta, allow to cool, and pour into a large mixing bowl. Gently fold all the vegetables and the tofu into the pasta.

Add all the dressing ingredients to a sealable container, seal, and shake it until the ingredients are thoroughly mixed. Pour over the cooked pasta and toss. Sprinkle ¼ cup of the shredded mozzarella cheese on top, then cover and chill for 1 hour.

Reverse Diet Potato and Egg Salad

Serves 8

6 hard-boiled eggs, sliced and chopped
8 large potatoes, cubed, with skin
1 8-ounce container fat-free sour cream
2 ounces tofu
1 tablespoon Dijon mustard
1 tablespoon minced garlic

   3   ribs celery, chopped small
   1   medium onion, chopped small
   paprika

Fill 2 medium saucepans with water ¾ full. Bring both pans to a boil, then add the eggs to one pan and the potatoes to the other. Cook the eggs for 15 minutes, then drain and place in cool water. Peel the cooled eggs and slice them. Boil the potatoes until they are just tender, then drain and run under cool water and set to the side. When the potatoes are cool, cut them into cubes.

In a side bowl, using a hand mixer on medium speed, blend the sour cream, tofu, Dijon mustard, and garlic until smooth and creamy.

In a large bowl mix the potatoes, eggs, celery, and onion and spoon in the creamy mixture. Mix everything and garnish with the paprika. Chill in the refrigerator for 1 hour or serve warm.

Reverse Diet Spinach, Strawberry, and Nut Salad

Serves 1

   2   cups fresh baby spinach leaves
  10   medium strawberries, sliced
   1   handful walnuts
   1   handful sliced almonds
   ½   cup chickpeas
   ½   cup fresh broccoli
   1   medium red onion, sliced thin
   black pepper to taste
   2   ounces fat-free raspberry vinaigrette dressing

Place the spinach leaves on a dinner plate, then add the strawberries, walnuts, almonds, chickpeas, broccoli, and onion. Sprinkle with the black pepper and toss. Place the dressing in a small container and use as dip.

SOUPS AND STEWS

Reverse Diet Veggie Soup

Serves 4

2 tablespoons low-fat, low-sodium butter substitute
3 tablespoons whole wheat all-purpose flour
2 cups low-sodium chicken stock
4 small potatoes, peeled and halved
1 teaspoon salt substitute
½ teaspoon ground black pepper
6 cups green onions, cut into 3-inch lengths
12 baby carrots
1 cup frozen corn
1½ pounds fresh green beans, cut into 1-inch lengths
2 cups frozen green peas

Make a roux by heating the butter substitute in a small saucepan and slowly stirring in the flour. Remove the mixture from the heat before it browns. Heat the stock to boiling in a medium pot; add the potatoes. Reduce the heat and simmer until the potatoes are tender, approximately 15 to 20 minutes.

Add the salt, pepper, onions, carrots, corn, and green beans; simmer until the vegetables are tender, then add the peas.

Stir the roux into the simmering vegetables. Cook, stirring constantly until the soup has boiled. Serve immediately.

Reverse Diet Tomato Soup

Serves 4

½ cup chopped onion
2 14½-ounce cans no-salt-added stewed tomatoes
½ cup egg noodles
2 tablespoons minced garlic
1 teaspoon parsley
½ teaspoon dried oregano
salt substitute and pepper to taste

In a large stockpot, brown the onion. Cook until the onion is tender. Stir in the stewed tomatoes, egg noodles, garlic, parsley, and oregano. Bring to a boil; reduce the heat, cover and simmer for 15 minutes, or until the noodles are tender. Season to taste with the salt and pepper. Serve hot.

Reverse Diet Southwestern Corn and Tomato Soup

Serves 2

2 cups low-sodium chicken stock
2 medium tomatoes, diced
½ cup corn
1 medium onion, sliced
1 cup frozen spinach

2 teaspoons minced garlic
¼ teaspoon chili pepper
½ teaspoon oregano
½ teaspoon parsley
2 tablespoons lemon juice

Purée all the ingredients in a blender. Add to a large pot over medium heat. Bring to a boil, then simmer for 15 to 20 minutes covered. Serve hot.

Reverse Diet Stew

Serves 4

butter-flavored cooking spray
1 pound lean beef sirloin
3 cups sliced raw potatoes
1½ cups chopped celery
2 cups sliced carrots
1 cup chopped onion
1½ cups frozen peas
1 can no-salt-added diced tomatoes
2 tablespoons minced garlic

In a large skillet sprayed with the cooking spray, brown the meat. Meanwhile, in a slow cooker, combine the potatoes, celery, carrots, onion, and peas. Spoon the browned meat into the cooker over the vegetables. In a small bowl, combine the tomatoes and garlic. Evenly pour the sauce into the cooker over the meat. Cover and cook on *low* for 6 to 8 hours. Mix well before serving.

Reverse Diet Spinach Vegetable Soup

Serves 4

4   cups water, divided
3   tablespoons converted brown rice, uncooked
¼   cup chopped onion
1   16-ounce package mixed frozen vegetables (broccoli, corn, red pepper)
½   cup frozen chopped spinach, thawed and drained
1½ cups seeded, chopped fresh tomatoes
2   tablespoons prepared salt substitute garlic herb seasoning blend
1½ teaspoons salt substitute
pepper to taste

Combine 2½ cups of the water and the rice and onion in a saucepan. Bring the mixture to a boil; reduce the heat. Simmer 15 minutes, then add the frozen vegetables.

Continue cooking 5 to 10 minutes or until the vegetables are cooked to desired doneness. Stir in the remaining water, spinach, fresh tomatoes, and seasoning blend. Season to taste with the salt substitute and pepper.

Reverse Diet French Onion Soup

Serves 4

1   pound onions, sliced
3   tablespoons unsalted butter substitute
3   cups low-sodium beef stock
3   teaspoons Worcestershire sauce
1   teaspoon thyme
2   tablespoons minced garlic

pinch ground black pepper
1   tablespoon salt substitute
4   slices whole wheat bread, toasted and cut into 4 pieces each
⅔   cup shredded low-fat Swiss cheese

Cook and stir occasionally the onions in the butter in a covered large saucepan over medium heat for 20 minutes until the onions are carmelized. Stir in the beef stock, Worcestershire sauce, thyme, garlic, black pepper, and salt substitute; heat to a boil. Remove from the heat.

Place the bread on a baking sheet; sprinkle the bread with the cheese. Broil 4 to 5 inches from the heat for about 1 minute or until the cheese is melted and golden.

Ladle the soup into bowls and top with bread.

Reverse Diet Creamy Asparagus Soup

Serves 4

4   cups diced asparagus
⅓   cup skim milk
½   cup fat-free sour cream
1   tablespoon Parmesan cheese
2   tablespoons cornstarch
pepper
parsley

Add the asparagus, milk, sour cream, and Parmesan cheese to a saucepan and bring to a boil on medium heat, stirring often. Cool the soup and pour into a blender and liquefy. Place the mixture back in the pan on medium heat.

In a separate cup or small container, add enough water to the cornstarch until a creamy mixture is formed, then add to the soup.

Bring to another boil, stirring constantly, then reduce the heat to a simmer. The soup will thicken as it cools.

Add pepper to taste, sprinkle with more Parmesan cheese, and garnish with the parsley.

Reverse Diet Clam Chowder

Serves 4

- 2 cups clam juice
- 1 cup water
- 1 pint shucked clams or two 6½-ounce cans of clams, low-sodium only, drained
- 2½ cups chopped and cubed potatoes
- 1 cup chopped onion
- 2 tablespoons minced garlic
- ¼ cup diced celery
- ½ teaspoon black pepper
- ¼ teaspoon parsley
- ½ cup tofu
- 1 teaspoon cornstarch
- 1 cup fat-free sour cream

In a large saucepan bring the clam juice and water to a boil. Add the clams, potatoes, onion, garlic, celery, black pepper, and parsley to the mixture. Bring back to a boil on high heat, then reduce the heat to medium. Cover and simmer 15 to 20 minutes, or until the potatoes are cooked to your liking. While the potatoes are cooking, in a medium bowl mix the tofu, cornstarch, and fat-free sour cream. Mix together with electric beaters on high until smooth. Add this mix to the soup mixture and turn the heat up until the soup comes to a low boil.

Reverse Diet Chicken Noodle Soup

Serves 4

4   cups low-sodium chicken stock
2   handfuls whole wheat wide-noodle pasta
1   chopped carrot
1   boneless and skinless chicken breast, filleted and cubed
olive oil
2   ribs celery, chopped
½   onion, diced
1   teaspoon minced garlic
½   teaspoon parsley
2   teaspoons rosemary
black pepper

Bring the chicken stock to a boil in a large saucepan and add the pasta and carrot. Boil the noodles according to the package directions. While cooking the noodles, place the chicken in a skillet brushed with the olive oil and sear. When the chicken is no longer pink, add it to the pasta and carrots along with the rest of the ingredients and stir together. Simmer until the vegetables are tender, about 10 more minutes. Serve hot.

SAUCES AND SEASONINGS

Reverse Diet Southern Barbecue Rub

Serves 4

2   tablespoons salt substitute
1   teaspoon dry mustard
1   tablespoon chili powder

- 1 tablespoon coarse black pepper
- 1 teaspoon cayenne pepper
- 2 tablespoons brown sugar
- 1 teaspoon thyme
- 1 teaspoon onion powder
- 2 tablespoons garlic powder
- 1 teaspoon parsley

Mix all the ingredients together in a bowl and rub or spread on your favorite protein.

Reverse Diet Caribbean Jerk Sauce

Serves 4

- 4 tablespoons lime juice
- 4 teaspoons thyme
- 1 tablespoon minced garlic
- ½ cup minced green onion
- 1 teaspoon cayenne pepper
- 1 tablespoon paprika
- 2 tablespoons light brown sugar
- ½ teaspoon cinnamon
- ½ teaspoon ginger
- 3 teaspoons allspice

Mix all the ingredients together in a bowl and rub or spread on your favorite protein.

Reverse Diet Sassy Salsa

Serves 4

- 4 tomatoes, diced small
- 1 medium onion, diced small
- 1 minced jalapeño pepper

½ red pepper, diced small
¼ teaspoon parsley
3 tablespoons chopped cilantro
¼ teaspoon black pepper
1 tomato, puréed
juice of 2 limes

Combine all the ingredients. Let stand in the refrigerator for at least 30 minutes. Serve with vegetables or chips.

Reverse Diet Quick Spaghetti Sauce

Serves 2

4 tomatoes, seeded and diced
1 onion, chopped
2 teaspoons olive oil
2 tablespoons minced garlic
1 teaspoon parsley
1 teaspoon oregano
2 tablespoons dry basil
¼ teaspoon chili powder
2 tablespoons Parmesan cheese
black pepper

In a large saucepan boil the tomatoes until they are soft, drain, and cool. When they are cooled, place them in a blender and run on medium until the desired consistency is achieved. Optional: You may also run them through a strainer to remove the seeds and skins.

In a skillet, brown the onion and pepper until they are slightly cooked. Add the tomatoes and spices to the onion and pepper mixture. Simmer over low heat, stirring constantly, until the vegetables are cooked down to the desired consistency. Sprinkle with the Parmesan cheese and pepper, and serve.

Reverse Diet Pesto Sauce

Serves 4

2   cups basil leaves, packed
½   cup Parmesan cheese
½   cup extra-virgin olive oil
5   cloves minced garlic
3   tablespoons pine nuts

Place all the ingredients in a blender and blend on medium speed for 2 to 3 minutes, scraping the sides occasionally.

Reverse Diet Honey Dijon Pizzazz Marinade

Serves 4

1   cup balsamic vinegar
2   tablespoons minced garlic
¼   cup no-sugar-added honey
⅓   cup lite Dijon mustard
1   teaspoon oregano
1   teaspoon parsley
½   teaspoon thyme
½   teaspoon rosemary
1   teaspoon basil
1   tablespoon Parmesan cheese
1   teaspoon black pepper
3   tablespoons lemon juice

Mix all the ingredients together in a bowl and pour over your favorite meats. Marinate 1 to 3 days.

Reverse Diet Cranberry Sauce

Serves 8

4   8-ounce bags cranberries
2   cups sugar substitute
1   teaspoon cinnamon
pinch clove

Cook the cranberries according to the package directions with the clove. When they are done, grind them, preferably in a rice grinder. In a large bowl, mix the cranberries and sugar substitute, and chill for about an hour. Before serving, sprinkle with the cinnamon.

Reverse Diet Barbecue Sauce

Serves 4

⅔   cup no-salt-added ketchup
3   tablespoons low-sodium soy sauce
1   medium onion, minced
2   tablespoons light brown sugar
¼   cup apple cider vinegar
2   tablespoons minced garlic
2   tablespoons light molasses
salt substitute to taste
black pepper to taste

In a medium-size saucepan, mix all the ingredients together and bring to a boil. Simmer over low heat until the mixture is thick, stirring occasionally.

DIPS AND SPREADS

Reverse Diet Apple and Tofu Dip with Assorted Fruit Platter

Serves 4 to 6

Dip

4	peeled and cored Delicious apples, sliced small
4	small strawberries
1	sliced peach
1	package firm tofu, drained and sliced
4	ounces fat-free sour cream
1	teaspoon vanilla extract
1	teaspoon cinnamon
1	teaspoon ginger
1	teaspoon nutmeg
1	tablespoon orange juice
½	tablespoon lemon juice
½	tablespoon sugar substitute

Platter

4	apples of your choice, sliced thin
2	kiwis, sliced thin
2	pears, sliced thin
2	peaches, sliced thin
1	cup pineapple, cubed
1	cup blueberries
1	cup strawberries
	mint sprigs

In a blender combine all the dip ingredients and blend until smooth. Pour into a deep bowl and place in the center of a serving platter. Arrange the fruit in alternating layers and garnish with the mint sprigs. Sprinkle with cinnamon.

Reverse Diet Spinach Dip

Serves 4 to 6

2 to 3 cups frozen or fresh spinach, cooked and drained
¼ teaspoon oregano
½ cup feta cheese
4 tablespoons minced garlic
6 ounces fat-free cream cheese, softened
1 serving tofu
¾ cup fat-free sour cream
salt substitute to taste
black pepper to taste

Preheat the oven to 350 degrees. Put all the ingredients in an oven-proof bowl and mix together. Bake for 25 minutes. Spoon into a separate bowl, set on a plate, and surround the dip with fresh vegetables of your choice.

Reverse Diet Tasty
Tofu Dip

Serves 1

½ cup tofu
1 tablespoon Parmesan cheese
2 tablespoons fat-free sour cream
2 tablespoons fat-free ranch dressing or your favorite fat-free salad dressing
½ teaspoon minced garlic
salt substitute to taste
black pepper to taste

In a small container, thoroughly mash all the ingredients together until smooth. Serve with your favorite vegetables or meats.

Reverse Diet Egg Salad Spread

Serves 4

6 hard-boiled eggs, chopped
6 tablespoons fat-free sour cream
¼ cup chopped celery
3 tablespoons finely chopped onion
1 tablespoon mustard, low-sodium
½ teaspoon celery seed
1 teaspoon minced garlic
½ tablespoon paprika
½ teaspoon cayenne pepper
salt substitute to taste
black pepper to taste

Mix all the ingredients together in a medium-size bowl and spread on your favorite low-calorie, low-sodium whole wheat bread, or use as a dip for vegetables.

Reverse Diet Olive Oil and Garlic Dip

Serves 1

2 tablespoons extra-virgin olive oil
2 teaspoons minced garlic
1 teaspoon parsley
1 teaspoon oregano
1 teaspoon basil
1 tablespoon Parmesan cheese

Mix all the ingredients together in a small bowl until thoroughly blended.

BEVERAGES

Reverse Diet Tangy Tofu Smoothie

Serves 1

1   serving tofu (see package)
½   cup blueberries
½   cup strawberries
2   slices pineapple
8   ounces orange juice
2   teaspoons low-fat yogurt
1   teaspoon sugar substitute
¼   teaspoon vanilla
½   cup ice

Add all the ingredients to a blender and blend until smooth and frothy.

Reverse Diet Sunshine Tea

Serves 1

8   ounces water
1   whole lemon or 4 tablespoons bottled lemon juice (with no sodium)

Optional

mint sprigs
1   teaspoon vanilla extract
sprinkle of cinnamon
1   teaspoon sugar substitute
½   teaspoon honey

Boil the water and add the lemon juice. Add any of the optional ingredients.

Reverse Diet Cranberry Crush

Serves 1

4   ounces no-sugar-added cranberry juice
4   ounces orange juice
¾   cup ice

Add all the ingredients to a blender and blend until smooth and frothy.

Reverse Diet Apple Smoothie

Serves 2

2   apples, peeled and cored
2   servings extra-firm tofu
5   ounces low-fat yogurt
1   cup orange juice
1   teaspoon cinnamon
1   teaspoon nutmeg
1   teaspoon mint
1   cup ice

Add all the ingredients in a blender and blend until smooth and frothy.

DESSERTS

Reverse Diet Sweet Potato Pie

Serves 4

Crust

2¾ cups water
⅔ cups cornmeal
2   tablespoon sugar substitute
½   teaspoon cinnamon
nonfat cooking spray

Filling

2   eggs
2   cups mashed sweet potatoes
½   cup sugar substitute
1   teaspoon cinnamon
½   teaspoon ginger
¼   teaspoon nutmeg
1   teaspoon vanilla extract
1½ cups skim milk
3   tablespoons light brown sugar

Bring the water to a boil, then add the cornmeal, sugar, and cinnamon slowly, stirring constantly. Lower the heat slightly, whisking the mixture until it is very thick, approximately 25 to 30 minutes. Spray a pie dish with the nonfat cooking spray, then pour the mixture into the dish. Place a sheet of waxed paper over the mixture and, using your fingers, spread the mix evenly in the dish.

Preheat the oven to 350 degrees. Mix the filling ingredients together and spoon the filling into the piecrust. Bake for 1 hour or until set. Let the pie cool and serve it warm or cold.

Reverse Diet Peach and Apple Mash

Serves 2

Mash

- ½ cup water
- 1 tablespoon cornstarch
- ½ cup orange juice
- 3 tablespoons light brown sugar
- 1 teaspoon cinnamon
- ¼ teaspoon nutmeg
- 1 teaspoon vanilla extract
- 1 teaspoon almond extract
- 3 medium peaches, pitted, with skins
- 2 large cooking apples, cored, with skins
- ½ cup pecans, crushed

Toppings

- ½ cup crushed shredded wheat
- ½ cup oatmeal
- 4 tablespoons honey

Preheat the oven to 400 degrees. In a large saucepan add the water, cornstarch, and orange juice. Bring the mixture to a boil, then add the rest of the mash ingredients and spices, stirring constantly until smooth.

Place all the ingredients in a baking dish, then smash them together with a potato masher. Add the toppings and bake in the center rack for 25 to 30 minutes.

Reverse Diet Island Pops

Serves 6

1 cup fresh strawberries
½ cup blueberries
2 peaches, peeled, pitted
½ cup orange juice
1 teaspoon lemon juice

Add all the ingredients to a blender and purée on high until smooth. Pour the mixture into popsicle trays and freeze for 1 to 2 days.

Reverse Diet Baked Apple

Serves 1

nonstick cooking spray
1 red apple, sliced in half, cored, peeled
cinnamon
ginger

Preheat the oven to 375 degrees. Spray a small cookie sheet with the nonstick cooking spray and place the apple halves face down on it. Sprinkle the apples with cinnamon and ginger and bake for 20 to 25 minutes or until the apples are soft in the middle.

Reverse Diet Banana Split

Serves 1

1   banana, sliced down the middle lengthwise
1   cup fat-free, sugar-free vanilla ice cream
3   pineapple slices
4   teaspoons pineapple juice, no-sugar-added
3   strawberries
3   tablespoons of fat-free, sugar-free whipped topping
¼   cup crushed walnuts

Place the banana in a dish and lay it open. Make 3 separate dollops of ice cream from 1 cup using a tablespoon. Put a pineapple ring on each dollop followed by a strawberry in the middle of each pineapple slice. Top off the banana split with the whipped cream and sprinkle the walnuts on top.

Reverse Diet Raspberry Delight

Serves 1

1½ cups fresh or frozen (thawed) raspberries
2   teaspoons cornstarch
½   cup fat-free, no-sugar-added ice cream, any flavor
2   tablespoons sliced almonds

Place the raspberries in a blender and purée until smooth. Press the raspberries through a sieve or cloth to the remove the seeds. Place the raspberries in a saucepan, add the cornstarch, and bring to a boil. Simmer for 15 minutes, stirring constantly. Let cool and chill for 1 to 2 hours.

Place the ice cream on a dessert plate. Pour the raspberry sauce over the ice cream and sprinkle the almonds on top.

Food Reality Check

Take a closer look at what you've been eating.

Foods	Serving Size	Calories	Fat (g)	Sodium (mg)
Boxed meals				
Betty Crocker Suddenly Salad, Classic Pasta	1½ cups	500	16	1,820
Mac & Cheese	1 cup	390	1.5	720
Betty Crocker Hamburger Helper	1 cup	310	24	880
Kraft Stove Top Stuffing Mix	2 ounces	360	2	500
Hungry Jack Au Gratin Potatoes	1 cup	300	2	1,140
Knorr-Lipton Pasta Sides	1 cup	270	2.5	650
Knorr-Lipton Asian Sides Chicken Fried Rice	1 cup	270	1.5	750
Top Ramen Noodles, Chicken	1 package	279	11	1,360
Healthy grain choices				
Whole wheat spaghetti	½ cup	180	1	0
Barilla PLUS multigrain enriched elbows	½ cup	200	1	25
Lentils, dried, cooked	½ cup	80	0	0
Brown rice, cooked	¾ cup	150	1	0
Barley, cooked	1 cup	193	1	5
Frozen foods				
Banquet Lasagna w/meat	1 cup	270	10	900
Banquet turkey and gravy mash	1	280	10	1,061
Banquet Pot Pie, beef	1 (7 ounces)	400	23	1,000
Green Giant Broccoli and Cheese Sauce	1 cup	113	4	807

Foods	Serving Size	Calories	Fat (g)	Sodium (mg)
Burritos, beef, bean, cheese	2 (10 ounces)	660	24	1,780
Hot Pockets, Chicken and Cheddar with Broccoli	1	602	22	1,303
Tater Tots	16 pieces	300	14	540
Onion rings, breaded	6	220	12	350
Healthier frozen foods				
Broccoli, plain	1 cup	50	0	44
Cauliflower	1 cup	34	0	32
Lima beans	½ cup	94	0	26
Carrots	½ cup	26	0	43
Blueberries, unsweetened	1 cup	78	0	1
Strawberries, unsweetened	1 cup	52	0	3
Miscellaneous				
La Choy Chow Mein	1 cup	108	2	1,135
Chinese takeout pork lo mein	1 cup	323	40	1,337
Chinese takeout egg rolls	2	280	30	1,020
Dairy				
Cottage cheese	½ cup	120	5	430
Velveeta Cheese	4 ounces	320	24	1,640
Healthier dairy choices				
Fat-free cottage cheese	½ cup	90	0	390
Part-skim mozzarella cheese	¼ cup	70	10	140
Reduced-fat Swiss cheese	1 slice	90	20	35
Provolone cheese	1 slice	70	5	120
Ricotta cheese, lite	¼ cup	60	3	55
Fat-free sour cream	2 tablespoons	20	0	40
Skim milk	1 cup	86	0	125
Fast food				
Burger King Double Whopper with cheese	1	1,070	70	1,500
French fries	1 large	500	25	880
Total Burger King meal	1	1,570	95	2,380
McDonald's Sausage Biscuit with Egg	1	446	28	932
McDonald's Hash Browns	1	130	8	330
Total McDonald's meal	1	576	36	1,262

Foods	Serving Size	Calories	Fat (g)	Sodium (mg)
KFC Original Recipe Chicken Breast	1	370	19	1,145
KFC Mashed Potatoes with Gravy	1	120	6	440
KFC Coleslaw	1	232	13	284
KFC biscuit	1	180	10	560
Total KFC meal	1	902	48	2,429
Papa John's Pizza, loaded	1 slice	405	20	1,114
Papa John's garlic sauce	1 serving	235	26	300
Total Papa John's meal	2 slices	1045	66	2,528

Healthier fast-food choices

Foods	Serving Size	Calories	Fat (g)	Sodium (mg)
Wendy's baked potato with broccoli	1 plain	310	0	25
Wendy's Grilled Chicken Breast sandwich	1 (2.9 ounces)	110	3	400
Wendy's Low-Fat Honey Mustard Dressing	1 teaspoon	25	0	40
Wendy's Side Salad, no dressing	1	60	3	160
Wendy's Deluxe Garden Salad, no dressing	1	110	6	320
Burger King Side Garden Salad, no dressing	1	25	0	15

Meats

Foods	Serving Size	Calories	Fat (g)	Sodium (mg)
Breaded fish filets	1 (2 ounces)	155	7	332
Breaded fish sticks	5	380	15	815
Chicken nuggets	5 pieces	230	16	470
Ham, center slice, country style	1 ounce	220	18	3,045
Hot dogs, beef and pork	1 (2 ounces)	183	17	639
Bacon	3 strips	156	12	714
Kielbasa	4 ounces	352	32	1,216
Sausage pork	5 links	240	20	840

Healthier protein choices

Foods	Serving Size	Calories	Fat (g)	Sodium (mg)
Chicken breast, no skin	6 ounces	284	2	36
Chicken thigh, no skin	1	113	5	49
Chicken leg, no skin	1 (3.3 ounces)	182	8	78
Chicken wings, baked, no skin	1	80	4	22
Turkey breast, no skin	5 ounces	238	7	99
Turkey dark meat, no skin	6 ounces	340	14	144
Lean pork loin	3 ounces	199	71	41

Foods	Serving Size	Calories	Fat (g)	Sodium (mg)
Cod	3 ounces	89	1	66
Salmon	3 ounces	155	7	48
Shrimp	8 large	44	0	98
Lean ground meat, broiled	3 ounces	231	74	65
Tofu	3 ounces	118	7	11
Deli meats				
Bologna	1 ounce	88	8	289
Salami, hard	2 slices	82	8	452
Pastrami	2 ounces	90	4	620
Smoked turkey breast	2.5 ounces	110	7	780
Smoked Virginia ham, 98% fat-free	2 slices	60	1	400
Canned foods				
Bush's Baked Beans	1 cup	240	2	1,100
Chickpeas	1 cup	285	3	718
Refried beans	1 cup	268	2	1,068
Green beans	1 cup	26	0	340
Corn	1 cup	132	2	792
Beets	1 cup	178	0	398
Black olives, jumbo, pitted	12	100	8	540
Green olives, medium-size	12	45	6	936
Sauerkraut	1 cup	44	0	1,560
Dill pickles	1 whole	10	0	660
Chef Boyardee Beef Ravioli 99% fat-free	1 cup	210	1	1,150
Healthier fresh food choices				
Chickpeas, dried, cooked	1 cup	269	4	11
Corn, yellow, cooked	1 cup	132	1	12
Beets	1 cup	72	0	77
Cabbage, cooked	1 cup	34	0	6
Cucumber	1 cup	14	0	2
Green beans, fresh, cooked	1 cup	44	0	4
Gravy made from mix				
Mushroom gravy	1 cup	70	1	1,402
Brown gravy	1 cup	75	2	1,076
Turkey gravy	1 cup	87	2	1,498
Pork gravy	1 cup	76	2	1,235

Foods	Serving Size	Calories	Fat (g)	Sodium (mg)
Sauces				
Teriyaki sauce	1 ounce	30	0	1,380
Del Monte cocktail sauce	¼ cup	100	0	910
Hunt's Spaghetti Sauce, Four Cheese	1 cup	100	2	1,200
Heinz Ketchup	1 tablespoon	15	0	190
Reverse Diet sauces				
Low-sodium ketchup	½ cup	35	0	10
Low-sodium cocktail sauce	½ cup	40	0	10
Low-sodium spaghetti sauce	1 cup	70	0	200
Low-sodium teriyaki sauce	1 ounce	10	0	300
Snacks				
Nachos Grande	6 to 8 (8.9 ounces)	568	31	1,800
Captain's Wafers, Cream Cheese and Chives	1 package	200	10	260
Cheese puffs	8 ounces	1,256	80	2,384
Cheetos	8 ounces	1,280	80	2,320
Pretzels	8 ounces	840	40	3,888
Chips, barbecue flavor	7 ounces	971	64	1,446
Tortilla, restaurant style	8 ounces	1,120	56	760
Wheat Thins	26	240	8	480
Oreos	2	107	5	147
Healthier snack choices				
Oatmeal or shredded wheat with orange juice	1 cup	300	1	1
Fat-free, sugar-free ice cream	½ cup	110	0	60
Baked tortillas, no sodium	18 chips	110	.5	5
Tofu tropical smoothie	8 ounces	140	7	11
Reverse Diet Nachos Grande	6 to 8 (8.9 ounces)	250	9	110

APPENDIX B

Calcium Sources

Confused by which form of calcium to choose? What matters most is consuming enough calcium. Calcium comes in many forms, including carbonate, citrate, gluconate, lactate, malate, phosphate, and amino acid chelates. The difference in absorption is minimal, but there is a difference in cost. Calcium carbonate is the most common and least expensive form. Do avoid calcium supplements from sources such as oyster shells, bone meal, or dolomite; these may contain large amounts of lead.

In a nutshell, select the sources you like, make sure they add up to a minimum of 800 to 1,500 milligrams, and *include them in your diet.*

FOOD SOURCES OF CALCIUM			
	Calcium (mg)	Carbohydrates (g)	Fat (g)
1 cup nonfat plain yogurt*	452	16	trace
1 cup low-fat plain yogurt*	415	16	2.3
1 cup low-fat fruit yogurt*	314	42	1.8
1 cup skim milk*	302	12	trace
1 cup whole milk*	291	12	8
1 cup 2% chocolate milk*	284	12	5
½ cup ice cream	88	16	7
½ cup frozen yogurt	89	20	1 (varies)
½ cup Edy's frozen yogurt	540	21	0
1 ounce Swiss cheese*	272	2	8
1 ounce cheddar cheese*	204	2	9
1 ounce mozzarella (part-skim)	183	1	5
1 ounce American cheese	174	0.5	9
1 ounce cottage cheese (2% fat)	77	8	4

	Calcium (mg)	Carbohydrates (g)	Fat (g)
½ cup tofu* (with calcium sulfate)	434	2	4
½ cup tofu	130	3	5
3 ounces sardines*	372	0	9
3 ounces salmon (canned)	167	0	5
3 ounces perch	117	0	1
¼ cup almonds	94	6	18
1 cup calcium-fortified orange juice* (Tropicana)	350	26	0
Propel fitness water	100	2	0
1 cup (8 ounces) Sanfaustino mineral water	100	0	0
1 packet Quaker Oatmeal for Women*	500	32	2.5
½ cup collard greens	152	5	2
½ cup mustard greens	138	5	2
½ cup turnip greens	99	5	2
½ cup broccoli	89	6	trace
½ cup okra	88	6	trace
½ cup kale	87	3	2
3.5 ounces wakame (seaweed), raw	150	9	1
3.5 ounces kelp (seaweed), raw	168	10	1

*These are excellent calcium sources.

Here is a brief review of popular supplements providing calcium. When taking supplements, it is best to split the dose of calcium throughout the day. More than 500 milligrams at one time is not as well absorbed.

POPULAR CALCIUM SUPPLEMENTS

Brand	# of pills to total 1,000-1,200 mg	Additional Ingredients
Caltrate 600 Plus	2	Vitamin D, magnesium, boron, copper, and zinc
Twinlab Bone Support	3	Magnesium and isoflavones
GNC Women's Daily Calcium Support	3	Vitamin D, magnesium, and silica (supposed to aid calcium utilization)
Vitamin Shoppe Osteo Protector	2	Vitamin D and magnesium
Schiff Bone Builder	3	Copper, silica, zinc, manganese, and vitamin K
Tums antacids, extra-strength	2	
Viactiv Soft Calcium chews	2	Vitamins D and K

Source: Women's Sports Medicine Center, New York, NY, 2002.

The Six Food Groups and Servings

Following is a breakdown of different calorie diets and recommended servings of each food group per diet. While we don't encourage counting calories, this chart will help you see how many vegetables, starches, and so on you'll need in your daily meals. In general, try to get your recommended food groups in each day, as appropriate to your true hunger levels and individual needs.

Calories	Starches (servings)	Vegetables (servings)	Fruits (servings)	Dairy (servings)	Fats (grams)	Proteins (ounces)
1,200	4	3	2	3	27-40	7
1,500	6	3	2	3	33-50	8
1,800	8	3	2	3	40-50	11
2,000	9	4	2	3	44-67	12
2,200	10	4	3	3	49-73	14

Average servings of the food groups are as follows:

Starches: 15 grams of carbohydrate per serving; 80 calories, 3 grams of protein, 0 to 1 gram of fat

½ cup cereal, grain, pasta, or starchy vegetables

⅓ cup of rice

1 ounce of bread, roll, etc.

¾ to 1 ounce of a snacklike product

Vegetables (nonstarchy): 5 grams of carbohydrate, 2 grams of protein; 25 calories

½ cup cooked vegetable or juice

1 cup raw

Fruits: 15 grams of carbohydrate per serving; 60 calories

1 small fresh fruit

½ cup canned fruit or fresh fruit or juice

¼ cup dried fruit

Dairy: 12 grams of carbohydrate, 8 grams of protein

1 cup milk

¾ cup plain yogurt

Fats: 5 grams of fat; 45 calories

1 teaspoon oil

6 to 10 nuts

1 tablespoon salad dressing

2 tablespoons reduced-fat salad dressing

1 tablespoon pumpkin or sunflower seeds

1 slice bacon

1 teaspoon butter

1 tablespoon cream cheese

2 tablespoons sour cream

3 tablespoons reduced-fat sour cream

Proteins: 0 carbohydrates, 7 grams of protein; 35 to 100 calories per ounce depending on selection and fat content

Source: The American Dietetic Association, *Lists for Weight Management*, 2005.

Index

additives, 67
all-or-nothing approach, 77, 125
apples
    Apple and Tofu Dip with
      Assorted Fruit Platter, 230
    Apple Smoothie, 234
    Baked, 237
    Peach and Apple Mash, 236
Artichoke Heart Casserole Medley,
    205
asparagus
    Creamy Asparagus Soup,
      223–224
    Fettucine and, 198-199
Asparagus, Fettucine and,
    198–199
aspartame, 165
attitude. *See* motivation

bacteria, friendly, 160
Baked Apple, 237
Banana Split, 238
Barbecue Sauce, 229
beans
    about, 159
    Refried, 215–216

beef
    in Stew, 221
    substitutions for, 163, 165
beverages
    about, 71–72
    Apple Smoothie, 234
    Cranberry Crush, 234
    Sunshine Tea, 72, 233
    Tangy Tofu Smoothie, 233
"Big Loser" parties, 183–184
bingeing, 98–99, 142–143. *See also*
    meal planning; motivation
blenders, 158
blood pressure, 74
blueberries, 160
body image, 21, 28–29
body type, 81–83
breakfast
    carbohydrates and, 81–82
    dinner foods for, 39–40, 82
    motivation and, 119
    skipping, 31
    See also individual recipes
Breakfast Wrap, 186–187
breast cancer, 157
breath freshener, 187

breathing exercise, 141–142
Bridge Phase, 123–124
  duration of, 167–168
  Food List do's and don't's,
    126–127
  journal for, 145–147
  menu plans, 129–137
  metabolism during, 125–126
  overeating during, 143–145
  reincorporating favorite foods,
    124–125, 127–129
  Reverse Buster, 142–143
  rewards during, 147–149
  sense of taste and, 138–142
broccoli
  about, 159
  Broccoli, Cauliflower, and
    Cheese, 214
Brown Rice and Tuna Casserole,
  204
buffets, 97–99
burgers
  about, 163
  Veggie, 187

cabbage, in Coleslaw, 214
caffeine, 72–74
calcium, 74, 75
calories
  caloric distribution, 7, 31, 40–41,
    81–83
  maintaining goal weight and,
    126
cancer, 157
carbohydrates, 69–70
  for breakfast, 81–82
  pasta, 70–71
Caribbean Jerk Sauce, 226

Cauliflower, Broccoli, and Cheese,
  214
celery
  about, 162
  Stuffed, 210
Cereal Mix, 76, 186
cheese
  Broccoli, Cauliflower, and, 214
  Mac and Cheese Bake, 196
chicken
  in Artichoke Heart Casserole
    Medley, 205
  Chicken and Tofu Stir Fry,
    203–204
  Chicken Noodle Soup, 225
  Clucky Chicken Pot Pie,
    201–202
  Italian, 197
  Jambalaya, 196–197
  Melt, 191
  Southern "Fried," 190–191
Chicken Melt, 191
Chili, 203
chili peppers, 160–161
cholesterol, 68, 160
Cinnamon Sauce, 212
Clam Chowder, 224
clothing
  after weight loss, 181–182
  for exercise, 154
Clucky Chicken Pot Pie, 201–202
cod, 161
Coleslaw, 214
condiments, 66, 109. *See also*
  sauces
containers
  for food preparation, 63
  for portion control, 108

cooking methods, 157–158. *See also* meal planning
Corn Bread, South of the Border Fiesta on, 215–216
cortisol, 41
Crabmeat, Stuffed Mushrooms with, 209
cranberry
    Crush, 234
    Sauce, 229
cravings, 35
    emotional eating and, 101
    taste changes and, 138–142
    triggers of, 35, 105–106, 145–147
    See also habits; motivation
Creamy Asparagus Soup, 223-224
cucumbers
    about, 162
    Delights, 210
Cunningham, Tricia, 1–5, 7

dairy, 159–160
    as food group, 38
    substitutions, 164
DASH diet (Dietary Advance to Stop Hypertension), 74
dehydration, 71–72
depression, 100
desserts
    Baked Apple, 237
    Banana Split, 238
    Island Pops, 237
    Peach and Apple Mash, 236
    Raspberry Delight, 238
    Sweet Potato Pie, 235
dips
    Apple and Tofu, 230

Egg Salad Spread, 232
    Olive Oil and Garlic Dip, 232
    Tasty Tofu, 231
drinks. *See* beverages

eating out
    avoiding take-out, 107
    buffets, 97–99
    healthy eating in restaurants, 108–111
egg
    Egg Bake, 200–201
    Salad Spread, 232
Eggplant Lasagna, 199–200
emotional eating
    rating emotions and, 46
    reframing negative thoughts and, 99–104
    sources of, 95
Enchiladas, Piggyback, 194–195
energy, caffeine and, 73
environmental distractions, 104–106
Equal, 165
erythritol, 165
estrogen, 157
exercise, 150–151
    benefits of, 151–153
    types of, 153–155
extra-virgin olive oil, 161

family members
    breakfast as family meal, 119
    Reverse Diet for, 107–108, 180–181, 183–184
fat, body, 151–153
fats, dietary
    as food group, 38

fats, dietary *(continued)*
  healthy substitutions for, 163,
    164
  olive oil, 161
  saturated fat, 68
  trans fat, 68
Fettucine and Asparagus,
  198–199
fish
  about, 161
  Brown Rice and Tuna Casserole,
    204
  Grumpy Grouper, 198
  Salmon Roly-Polies, 211
  Simply Salmon, 192
  Stuffed Tuna Tofu Tomatoes,
    188–189
  See also seafood
flour, 165
food choices
  cravings and, 35, 101, 105–106,
    138–142, 145–147
  experimenting with new foods,
    155–157
  high-octane reverse foods,
    158–162
  reincorporating favorites,
    124–125, 127–129
food groups, 37–39
food labels, 66–68
  example, 68
  serving sizes and, 82
Food Lists
  for Bridge Phase, 126–127
  for Weight-Loss Phase, 32–35
French Onion Soup, 222–223
Fried Zucchini, 212–213
frozen foods, 108

fruits
  as alternative to sweets, 76
  as food group, 38
  as high-octane reverse food,
    159–162
  Island Pops, 237
  Tangy Tofu Smoothie, 233
  See also individual names of fruits

gardening, 162
garlic
  about, 160
  Olive Oil and Garlic Dip, 232
goals
  achievement of, 175
  for Bridge Phase, 145–147
  for exercise, 154–155
  for habit change, 27–29
  for health, 20–24, 26–27
  long-term, 117–118
  for Maintenance Phase, 179
  motivation and, 115–119
  realistic vs. idealistic weight,
    20–24, 26–27
  short-term, 117–119
  for Weight Loss Phase, 17–18
Good Morning America (ABC-TV),
  7, 8
grains
  as food group, 38
  as high-octane reverse food, 159
  See also individual recipes
grapes, 160
green tea, 74
Grilled Fruit Kabob with Cinnamon Sauce, 211–212
grocery shopping, 62, 162. *See also*
  meal planning

Grouper, Grumpy, 198
Grumpy Grouper, 198

habits
  benefits of Reverse Diet and,
    19–20
  cravings and, 35, 101, 105–106,
    138–142, 145–147
  developing healthy eating
    patterns, 92
  emotional eating as, 101
  goals for, 27–29
  mindful attention to, 86–87
  overeating and, 47, 96–97
hamburgers, 163
herbs
  growing, 162
  Pesto Sauce, 228
high-risk moments, 89–92,
    98–99, 145–147. *See also*
    cravings; motivation;
    overeating
holiday meals, 112–113
Honey Dijon Pizzazz Marinade,
    228
hormones
  cortisol, 41
  estrogen, 157
Hunger Scale, 41–46, 82
hydration, 71–72
hypertension, 74

iceberg lettuce, 162
ice cream, 164
*International Journal of Eating
  Disorders,* 101
Island Pops, 237
Italian Chicken, 197

Jambalaya, 196–197
jerks. *See* sauces
journal, 24
  for Diet Bridge Phase, 145–147
  goal setting exercises, 25–27,
    28–29, 175, 179
  meal planning exercises, 66, 129
  motivation exercises, 89, 98–99,
    102–103, 118
  portion control exercises, 80–81,
    86–87
  template, 45
*Journal of the American Dietetic
  Association,* 79

kids' restaurant meals, 110
kitchen
  appliances, 157–158
  stocking, 106–108

lasagna
  about, 163
  Eggplant, 199–200
lean mass, 84, 150–155
lettuce, 162
"life pie," 24–26, 177–179
lifestyle. *See* habits

Mac and Cheese Bake, 196
main courses
  Artichoke Heart Casserole Med-
    ley, 205
  Breakfast Wrap, 186–187
  Brown Rice and Tuna Casserole,
    204
  Cereal Mix, 76, 186
  Chicken and Tofu Stir Fry,
    203–204

main courses *(continued)*
 Chicken Melt, 191
 Chili, 203
 Clucky Chicken Pot Pie, 201–202
 Egg Bake, 200–201
 Eggplant Lasagna, 199–200
 Fettucine and Asparagus,
  198–199
 Grumpy Grouper, 198
 Italian Chicken, 197
 Jambalaya, 196–197
 Mac and Cheese Bake, 196
 Meat Loaf, 195
 Piggyback Enchiladas, 194–195
 Rice Cake Pizza, 193–194
 Scallops with Linguini in
  Tomato and Basil Sauce, 206
 Shrimp a la Queen, 193
 Simply Salmon, 192
 Sloppy Toms, 191–192
 Southern "Fried" Chicken,
  190–191
 Southern Shrimp Creole,
  189–190
 Stuffed Green Peppers, 188
 Stuffed Tuna Tofu Tomatoes,
  188–189
 Stuffed Zucchini, 207
 Veggie Burger, 187
Maintenance Phase, 167, 171–175
 excessive weight loss and,
  175–176
 identity and, 179–181
 "life pie" priorities and, 177–179
 lifestyle changes and, 176–177
 rewards for, 181–184
maltitol, 165
marinades. *See* sauces

meal planning
 all-or-nothing approach and, 77,
  125
 alternatives to sweets, 76
 caffeine and, 72–74
 calcium and, 75
 carbohydrates in, 69–71
 checking food labels for,
  66–68
 cooking methods and, 157–158
 for holidays, 112–113
 hydration and, 71–72
 Maintenance Phase and,
  173–174
 menu plans, Bridge Phase,
  129–137
 menu plans, Weight-Loss Phase,
  36–37, 51–61
 motivation and, 106–108
 nuts and, 74
 processed foods and, 64–66
 for restaurants, 108–111
 shopping and, 49–50, 61–64
 sodium and, 75–77
 Sunshine Tea and, 72
 time of preparation, 63
 tips for, 77
 for vacations, 111–112
 for workplace, 93–95
 See also individual recipes
meat, buying, 63. *See also individual types of meat*
Meat Loaf, 195
menus
 Bridge Phase, 129–137
 Reverse Buster, 143
 Weight-Loss Phase, 36–37, 51–61
 See also individual recipes

metabolism, 31, 39–40, 125–126.
    See also calories
microwave ovens, 157–158
milk, 38. *See also* dairy
milkshakes, 164
mindfulness
    breathing technique for,
        141–142
    habits and, 86–87
    negative thoughts and, 28–29,
        99–104
motivation, 88–89
    breakfast and, 119–120
    buffets and, 97–99
    eating out and, 108–111
    emotional obstacles to, 99–102
    environmental distractions and,
        104–106
    for exercise, 155
    goals and, 115–119
    high-risk moments and, 89–92,
        98–99, 145–147
    holidays and, 112–113
    journal for, 145–147
    kitchen set-up and, 106–108
    negative thoughts and, 102–104
    overeating and, 92–93, 96–97
    support system and, 114–115
    vacationing and, 111–112
    for weight loss, 113
    work stress and, 93–95
muscle, 84, 150–155
mushrooms
    about, 160
    Stuffed, with Crabmeat, 209

National Registry of Weight
    Control, 151

negative thoughts
    awareness of, 99–102
    reframing, 28–29, 102–104
normalizing, of foods, 101
Nutrasweet, 165
nuts
    about, 74, 161
    Spinach, Strawberry, and Nut
        Salad, 218–219

oatmeal
    about, 159
    in Tricia's Special Cereal, 76,
        186
olive oil
    about, 161
    Olive Oil and Garlic Dip, 232
onions
    about, 161
    French Onion Soup, 222–223
orange juice, 158–159
osteoporosis, 75
overeating
    alternatives to, 92–93
    during Bridge Phase, 127–129,
        140–141, 143–145
    identifying behavior of, 96–97
    See also motivation

parsley, 162
pasta
    about, 70–71, 163, 164
    Chicken Noodle Soup, 225
    Fettucine and Asparagus,
        198–199
    Mac and Cheese Bake, 196
    Quick Spaghetti Sauce, 227
    Salad, 216–217

pasta *(continued)*
Scallops with Linguini in
Tomato and Basil Sauce, 206
Peach and Apple Mash, 236
peppers
chili, 160–161
Stuffed Green Peppers, 188
personal trainers, 155
Pesto Sauce, 228
physical activity. *See* exercise
Piggyback Enchiladas, 194–195
pizza
about, 163
Rice Cake Pizza, 193–194
plateaus, weight, 84–87
pork, in Piggyback Enchiladas,
194–195
portion control, 9, 78
body composition and, 84
during Bridge Phase, 127–129,
139–142
containers for, 108
Hunger Scale and, 41–46, 82
individual needs and, 81–83
mindful attention and, 86–87
motivation and, 101–102
for pasta, 70–71
portion distortion, 78–81
restaurant meals and, 110
USDA examples, 82–83
weighing schedule and, 83–84
weight plateau and, 84–86
potatoes
and Egg Salad, 217–218
Scalloped, 213
Sweet Potatoes, 209
Sweet Potato Pie, 235
Twice-Stuffed, 208

preservatives, 67
prioritizing, 24–26, 177–179
processed foods, 64–66
proteins
carbohydrates and, 69–70
as food group, 38

Quick Spaghetti Sauce, 227

Raspberry Delight, 238
recipes
beverages, 233–234
desserts, 235–238
dips and spreads, 230–232
main courses, 186–207
salads, 216–219
sauces, 225–229
side dishes, 208–216
soups and stews, 219–225
Tricia's Special Cereal, 76, 186
Refried Beans, 215–216
relationships, Maintenance Phase
and, 177–178
relaxation exercise, 141–142
residual hunger, 40–41. *See also*
calories
restaurants
avoiding take-out, 107
buffets, 97–99
healthy eating in, 108–111
Reverse Buster, 142–143
Reverse Diet
benefits of, 19–20, 177–178
cooking methods for, 157–158
development of, 1–8
exercise and, 150–155
for family members, 107–108,
180–181, 183–184

habits and, 27

high-octane reverse foods for, 158–162

journal for, 24

"life pie," 24–26, 177–179

lifestyle change, 18–19

new foods for, 155–157

phases of, 11–13 (*See also* Bridge Phase; Maintenance Phase; Weight-Loss Phase)

premise of, 9–11

Reverse Diet moments, 27–29, 140, 180

substitutions for favorite recipes, 163–168

See also goals

Reverse Diet Bridge. *See* Bridge Phase

Reverse Diet Club, 114

Reverse Moments, 27–29, 140, 180

rewards

  for Bridge Phase, 147–149

  for Maintenance Phase, 181–184

Rice and Tuna Casserole, 204

Rice Cake Pizza, 193–194

ring test, 75–76

romaine lettuce, 162

saccharin, 165

salads

  Pasta, 216–217

  Potato and Egg, 217–218

  Spinach, Strawberry, and Nut, 218–219

salmon, 161

  Roly-Polies, 211

  Simply Salmon, 192

salt. *See* sodium

Sassy Salsa, 226–227

saturated fat, 68

sauces

  Barbecue, 229

  Caribbean Jerk, 226

  Cinnamon, 212

  Cranberry, 229

  Honey Dijon Pizzazz Marinade, 228

  Pesto, 228

  Quick Spaghetti, 227

  Sassy Salsa, 226–227

  Tomato and Basil, 206

Scalloped Potatoes, 213

Scallops with Linguini in Tomato and Basil Sauce, 206

seafood

  Clam Chowder, 224

  Jambalaya, 196–197

  Mushrooms with Crabmeat, 209

  Scallops with Linguini in Tomato and Basil Sauce, 206

  Shrimp a la Queen, 193

  See also fish

serving sizes, 82. *See also* portion control

shopping, 49–50, 61–66, 162. *See also* meal planning

shredded wheat

  about, 159

  Tricia's Special Cereal, 76, 186

shrimp

  in Jambalaya, 196–197

  a la Queen, 193

  Southern, Creole, 189–190

side dishes

  Broccoli, Cauliflower, and Cheese, 214

side dishes *(continued)*
  Coleslaw, 214
  Cucumber Delights, 210
  Fried Zucchini, 212–213
  Grilled Fruit Kabob with
    Cinnamon Sauce, 211–212
  Salmon Roly-Polies, 211
  Scalloped Potatoes, 213
  South of the Border Fiesta on
    Corn Bread, 215–216
  Stuffed Celery, 210
  Stuffed Mushrooms with
    Crabmeat, 209
  Sweet Potatoes, 209
  Twice-Stuffed Potatoes, 208
Simply Salmon, 192
Skolnik, Heidi, 6–8
sleep, 41
Sloppy Toms, 191–192
sodium, 66–67
  substitutes, 164
  water weight and, 75–76
sorbitol, 165
soups/stews
  about, 71
  Chicken Noodle, 225
  Clam Chowder, 224
  Creamy Asparagus, 223-224
  French Onion, 222–223
  Southwestern Corn and Tomato,
    220
  Spinach Vegetable, 222
  Stew, 221
  Tomato, 220
  Veggie, 219
Southern Barbecue Rub, 225–226
Southern "Fried" Chicken,
    190–191

Southern Shrimp Creole,
    189–190
South of the Border Fiesta on
    Corn Bread, 215–216
Southwestern Corn and Tomato
    Soup, 220
soy foods, 156–157
spaghetti, 164. *See also* pasta
spinach
  about, 159
  Dip, 231
  Strawberry, and Nut Salad with,
    218–219
  Vegetable Soup with, 222
Splenda, 165
starches, 70, 79–80. *See also*
    carbohydrates
steak, 163–164
Stew, 221. *See also* soups/stews
strawberries
  about, 162
  Spinach, Strawberry, and Nut
    Salad, 218–219
strength training, 153–154
stress
  high-risk moments, 89–92,
    98–99, 145–147
  identifying, 96–97
  at work, 93–95
Stuffed Celery, 210
Stuffed Green Peppers, 188
Stuffed Mushrooms with Crab-
    meat, 209
Stuffed Tuna Tofu Tomatoes,
    188–189
Stuffed Zucchini, 207
substitutions
  for favorite recipes, 163–168

for restaurant foods, 109
sucralose, 165
sugar
  about, 67
  alcohols, 165
  substitutes, 164
Sunshine Tea
  recipe, 233
  uses for, 72
support system
  friends for, 114–115
  Reverse Diet Club as, 114
Sweet 'N Low, 165
sweet potatoes
  Pie, 235
  as side dish, 209
sweets, alternatives to, 76

tacos
  Beef, 165
  Turkey, 166
take-out food, 107, 110. *See also*
  restaurants
Tangy Tofu Smoothie, 233
taste, 138–142
Tasty Tofu Dip, 231
tea
  green tea, 74
  Sunshine Tea, 72, 233
tofu, 156–157
  Apple and Tofu Dip, 230
  in Apple Smoothie, 234
  in Breakfast Wrap, 186–187
  in Brown Rice and Tuna
    Casserole, 204
  Chicken and Tofu Stir Fry,
    203–204
  in Clam Chowder, 224

in Potato and Egg Salad, 217
in Rice Cake Pizza, 193–194
in Scalloped Potatoes, 213
in Spinach Dip, 231
Stuffed Tuna Tofu Tomatoes,
  188–189
Tangy Tofu Smoothie,
  233
Tasty Tofu Dip, 231
in Veggie Burger, 187
tomatoes, 160
  Quick Spaghetti Sauce, 227
  Southwestern Corn and Tomato
    Soup, 220
  Stuffed Tuna Tofu Tomatoes,
    188–189
  Tomato Soup, 220
  Veggie Soup, 219
trans fat, 68
Tricia's Special Cereal, 76, 186
tuna
  Brown Rice and Tuna Casserole,
    204
  Stuffed Tuna Tofu Tomatoes,
    188–189
turkey
  about, 163
  in Chili, 203
  in Meat Loaf, 195
  in Sloppy Toms, 191–192
  in Stuffed Zucchini, 207
  Tacos, 166
Twice-Stuffed Potatoes, 208

U.S. Department of Agriculture
  (USDA), 82–83

vacations, meals for, 111–112

vegetables
   as food group, 38
   growing, 162
   as high-octane reverse food,
      159–162
   *See also individual vegetable
      names and recipes*
vegetarian/vegan diets, 34–35
Veggie Burger, 187
Veggie Soup, 219

water, 71–72
water weight
   carbohydrates and, 70
   Reverse Buster for, 142–143
   ring test and, 75–76
weighing
   body composition and, 84
   schedule for, 83–84, 144
   weight plateau and, 84–87
weight loss, 113
   caffeine and, 73
   excessive, 175–176
   exercise for, 150–155
   realistic vs. idealistic goals,
      20–24, 26–27
   See also motivation; Weight-Loss
      Phase
Weight-Loss Phase, 167
   basics, 30–31
   calorie distribution, 31, 40–41
   dinner foods at breakfast, 39–40

food group combinations,
   37–39
Food List, 32–35
Hunger Scale and, 41–46, 82
journal for, 43–47
menus, 36–37, 51–61
portion control and, 79–87
tips for, 47–48
See also meal planning; Reverse
   Diet
weight training, 152
wheat
   shredded wheat, 159
   Tricia's Special Cereal, 76,
      186
whole foods, 64–66
   processed foods vs., 65
   taste and, 138–142
whole wheat pasta, 70–71
workplace
   schedule, 48
   stress and, 93–95
Wrap, Breakfast, 186–187

xylitol, 165

yogurt, 38, 159–160
yo-yo dieting, 1–3, 28, 152

zucchini
   Fried, 212–213
   Stuffed, 207